ZERO POINT WEIGHT LOSS COOKBOOK

Elevating Your Weight Loss Journey With Flavor

Daniel S. Yoon

Table Of Contents

Copyright

Introduction

Welcome to the culinary revolution of 2024, where healthy eating meets culinary delight in our comprehensive "2024 Zero Point Weight Loss Cookbook". In this innovative collection, we present an array of mouthwatering recipes meticulously crafted to support your weight loss journey while tantalizing your taste buds. Harnessing the power of zero point ingredients, each recipe is thoughtfully designed to help you achieve your wellness goals without sacrificing flavor or satisfaction. this cookbook is your ultimate guide to embracing a healthier lifestyle without compromising on taste.

Grilled Cilantro Lime Shrimp Kebabs

**Prep time: 25 minutes
Cook time: 5 minutes
Servings: 1**

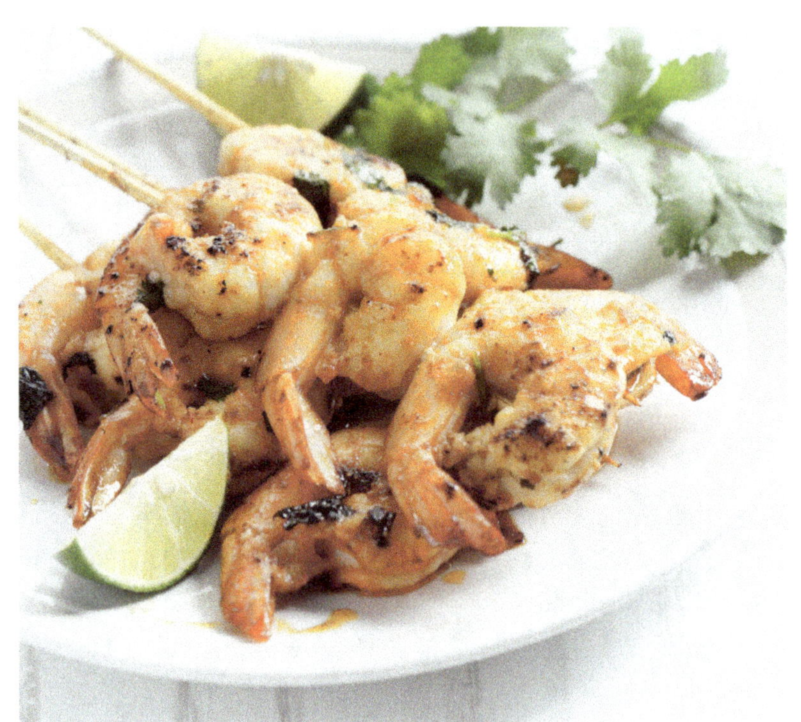

Ingredients:

- pound large shrimp, peeled and deveined
- 1/4 cup chopped fresh cilantro
- Zest and juice of 1 lime
- 2 cloves garlic, minced
- 2 tablespoons olive oil

Procedure:

- In a bowl, combine chopped fresh cilantro, lime zest, lime juice, minced garlic, olive oil, ground cumin, paprika, salt, and pepper to create the marinade. Mix well.
- Add the peeled and deveined shrimp to the marinade, ensuring they are evenly coated. Let them marinate in the refrigerator for at least 30 minutes, or up to 2 hours for more flavor.

3

- 1/2 teaspoon ground cumin
- 1/2 teaspoon paprika
- Salt and pepper to taste

- If you're using wooden skewers, soak them in water for at least 30 minutes to prevent burning.
- Preheat the grill to medium-high heat.
- Thread the marinated shrimp onto the skewers, alternating with slices of bell peppers, onions, or any other desired vegetables.
- Place the shrimp kebabs on the preheated grill and cook for 2-3 minutes on each side, or until the shrimp are pink and opaque.
- Once cooked, remove the shrimp kebabs from the grill and serve immediately.

Nutritional information

- Serving: 1
- Calories: 74 kcal
- Carbohydrates: 3g,
- Protein: 13g
- Fat: 1g
- Cholesterol: 94 mg
- Sodium: 384 mg
- Fiber: 1g

Turkey Pumpkin Chili

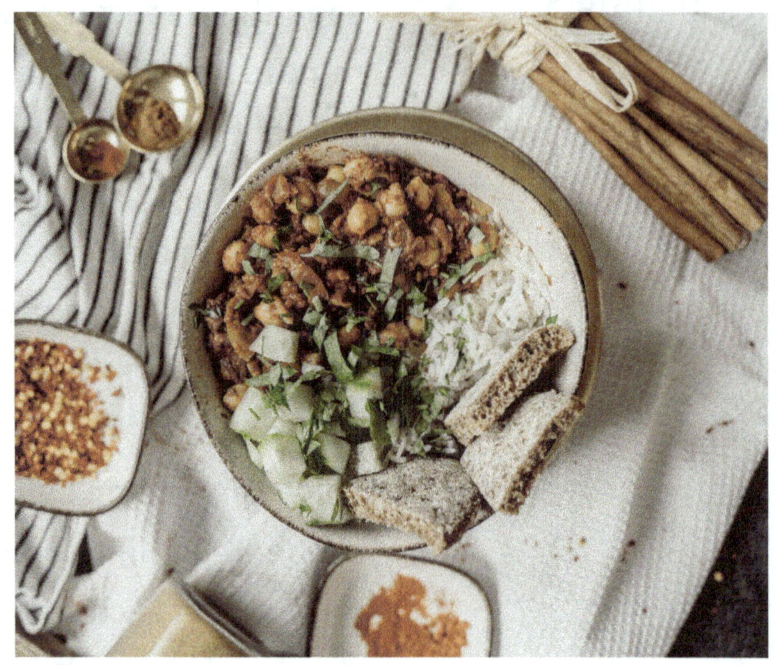

Prep time: 20 minutes
Cook time: 1 hr

Servings: 1

Ingredients:

- 1 tablespoon olive oil
- 1 onion, chopped
- 3 cloves garlic, minced
- 1 pound ground turkey
- 1 can (15 ounces) pumpkin puree
- 1 can (15 ounces) diced tomatoes, undrained

Procedure:

- Heat the olive oil in a large pot or Dutch oven over medium heat. Add the diced onion and bell pepper, and cook until softened, about 5 minutes.
- Add the minced garlic to the pot and cook for an additional minute until fragrant.
- Add the ground turkey to the pot, breaking it apart with a spoon, and cook until browned and cooked through, about 6-8 minutes.
- Once the turkey is cooked, add the pumpkin puree, diced tomatoes, black beans, kidney beans, and chicken or vegetable broth to the pot. Stir to combine.

- 1 can (15 ounces) black beans, drained and rinsed
- 1 can (15 ounces) kidney beans, drained and rinsed
- 1 cup chicken or vegetable broth
- 1 tablespoon chili powder
- 1 teaspoon ground cumin
- 1 teaspoon dried oregano
- 1/2 teaspoon ground cinnamon
- Salt and pepper .

- Season the chili with chili powder, ground cumin, paprika, cinnamon, salt, and pepper. Stir well to incorporate the spices.
- Bring the chili to a simmer, then reduce the heat to low. Cover and let the chili simmer for about 20-25 minutes, stirring occasionally.
- After simmering, taste the chili and adjust the seasoning if needed.
- Serve the Turkey Pumpkin Chili hot, topped with shredded cheese, sour cream, chopped cilantro, sliced green onions.

Nutritional information

- Calories: 250kcal
- Carbohydrates: 37g
- Protein: 24g
- Fat: 2g
- Cholesterol: 31mg
- Sodium: 941mg
- Potassium: 1183mg
- Fiber: 12g
- Sugar: 11g
- Vitamin C: 35mg
- Calcium: 132mg
- Iron: 6mg

Spicy Tortilla Chips

Prep time: 3 minutes
Cook time: 10 minutes
Servings: 4

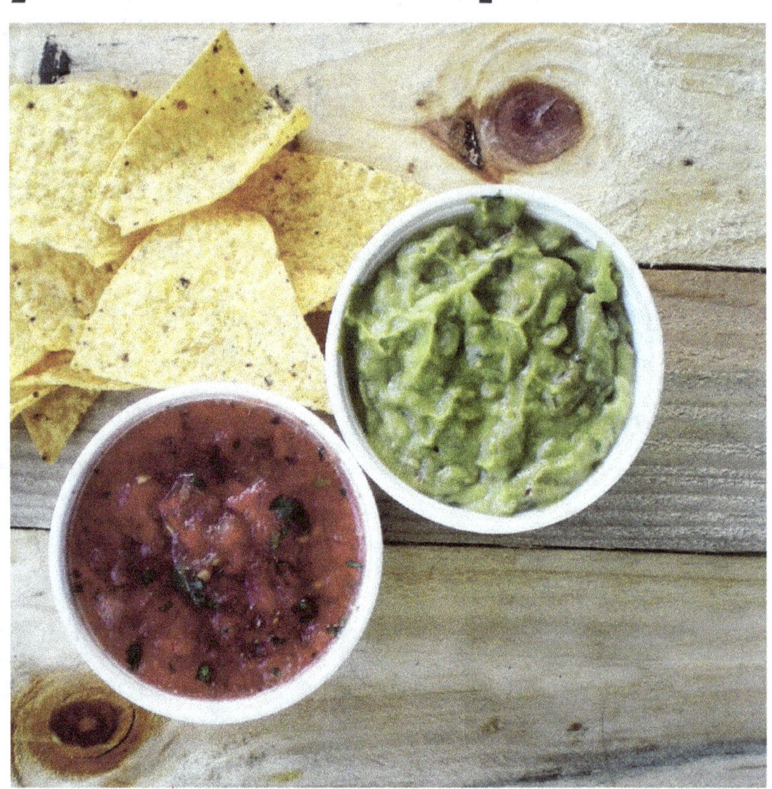

Ingredients:

- pound large shrimp, peeled and deveined
- 1/4 cup chopped fresh cilantro
- Zest and juice of 1 lime
- 2 cloves garlic, minced
- 2 tablespoons olive oil

Procedure:

- In a bowl, combine chopped fresh cilantro, lime zest, lime juice, minced garlic, olive oil, ground cumin, paprika, salt, and pepper to create the marinade. Mix well.
- Add the peeled and deveined shrimp to the marinade, ensuring they are evenly coated. Let them marinate in the refrigerator for at least 30 minutes, or up to 2 hours for more flavor.
- If you're using wooden skewers, soak them in water for at least 30 minutes to prevent burning.

7

- 1/2 teaspoon ground cumin
- 1/2 teaspoon paprika
- Salt and pepper to taste

- Preheat the grill to medium-high heat.
- Thread the marinated shrimp onto the skewers, alternating with slices of bell peppers, onions, or any other desired vegetables.
- Place the shrimp kebabs on the preheated grill and cook for 2-3 minutes on each side, or until the shrimp are pink and opaque.
- Once cooked, remove the shrimp kebabs from the grill and serve immediately.

Nutritional information

- Serving: 1
- Calories: 74 kcal
- Carbohydrates: 3g,
- Protein: 13g
- Fat: 1g
- Cholesterol: 94 mg
- Sodium: 384 mg
- Fiber: 1g

Buffalo Chicken Celery Bites

Prep time: 5 minutes
Cook time: 5 minutes
Servings: 4

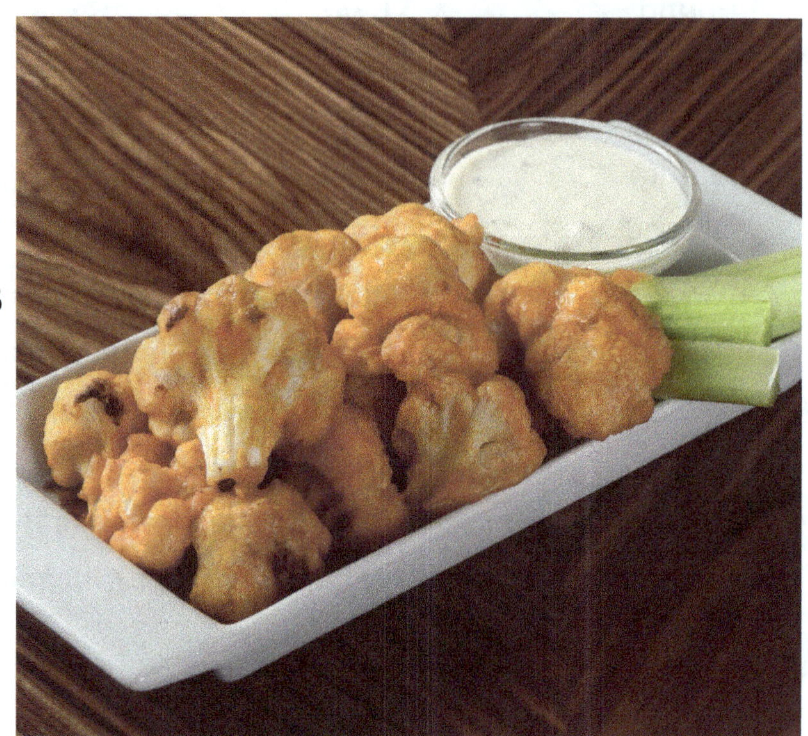

Ingredients:

- 4-6 celery stalks, washed and trimmed
- 1 cup cooked and shredded chicken
- 1/4 cup buffalo sauce
- 2 tablespoons mayonnaise or Greek yogurt

Procedure:

- In a mixing bowl, combine the shredded chicken, buffalo sauce, mayonnaise or Greek yogurt, chopped green onions or chives, salt, and pepper. Mix well until everything is evenly combined and coated in the buffalo sauce mixture.

- Taste the buffalo chicken mixture and adjust the seasoning.

9

- 1 tablespoon chopped green onions or chives
- Salt and pepper.

- Slice the celery stalks into bite-sized pieces, each about 3-4 inches long.
- Spoon a small amount of the buffalo chicken mixture onto each celery piece, filling the hollow center.
- Arrange the filled celery bites on a serving platter and serve immediately.
- Enjoy your delicious and spicy Buffalo Chicken Celery Bites as a snack or appetizer!

Nutritional information

- Calories: 80Kcal
- Total Fat: 1g
- Fat: 1g
- Cholesterol: 39mg
- Sodium: 92mg
- Total Carbohydrate:3g
- Dietary Fiber: 1g
- Sugars: 1g
- Protein 13g

Hummus

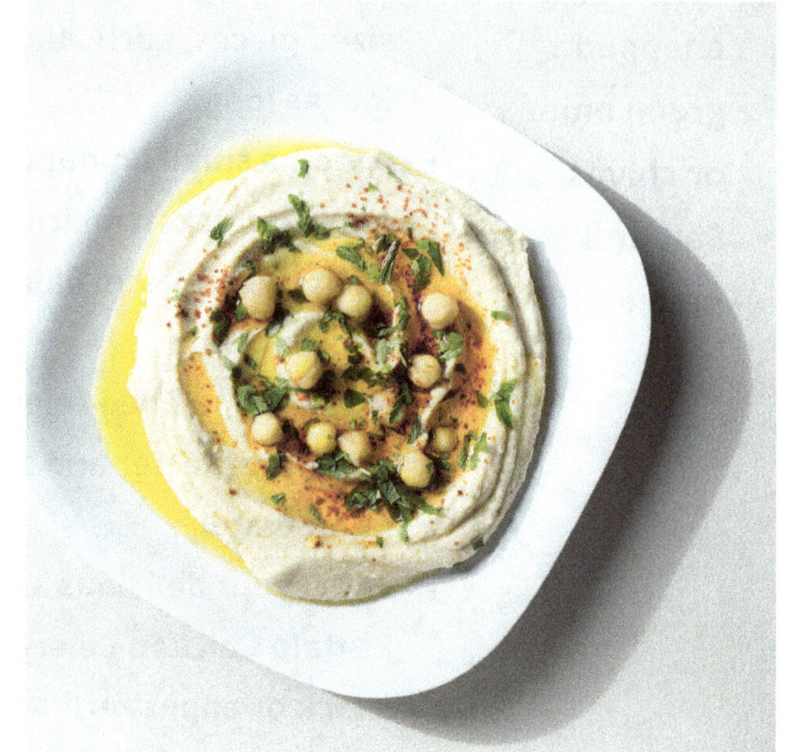

Ingredients:

- 1 can (15 ounces) chickpeas (garbanzo beans), drained and rinsed
- 2-3 tablespoons tahini (sesame seed paste)

Procedure:

- In a food processor, combine the drained and rinsed chickpeas, tahini, olive oil, minced garlic, lemon juice, ground cumin, and a pinch of salt.
- Process the mixture until smooth and creamy, scraping down the sides of the food processor bowl . If the hummus is too thick, you can add 2-4 tablespoons of water, one tablespoon at a time, until you reach your desired consistency.

11

- 2 tablespoons extra virgin olive oil
- 2 cloves garlic, minced
- Juice of 1 lemon
- 1/2 teaspoon ground cumin
- Salt to taste
- 2-4 tablespoons water

- Taste the hummus and adjust the seasoning if needed, adding more salt or lemon juice
- Once the hummus is smooth and creamy, transfer it to a serving bowl.
- Drizzle a little extra virgin olive oil over the top of the hummus and sprinkle with paprika, chopped fresh parsley, or toasted pine nuts for added flavor and garnish.
- Serve the hummus with pita bread, fresh vegetables, or crackers for dipping.

Nutritional information

- Calories: 70kcal
- Fat: 4g
- Carbohydrates: 6g
- Protein: 3g
- Fiber: 2g
- Sodium: 100mg

Yoghurt Chicken

Prep time: 10 minutes
Cook time: 20 minutes

Servings: 5

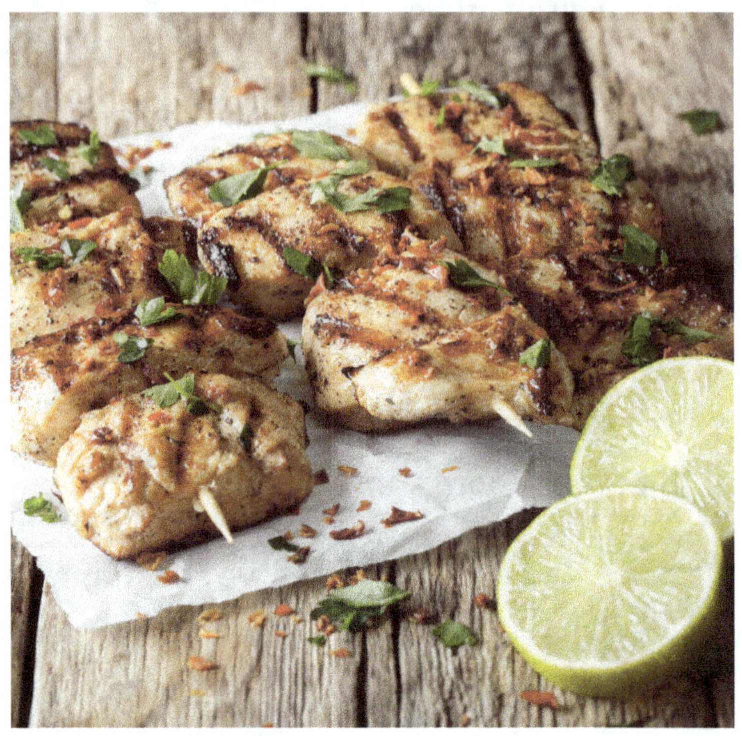

Ingredients:

- 4 boneless, skinless chicken breasts
- 1 cup plain Greek yogurt
- 2 tablespoons olive oil
- 2 cloves garlic, minced
- 1 tablespoon lemon juice

Procedure:

- In a mixing bowl, combine the plain Greek yogurt, olive oil, minced garlic, lemon juice, paprika, ground cumin, ground coriander, ground turmeric, salt, and pepper. Mix well to combine and create the marinade.

- Place the chicken breasts in a shallow dish or a resealable plastic bag. Pour the yogurt marinade over the chicken, ensuring that each piece is coated evenly. Marinate the chicken in the refrigerator for at least 30 minutes, or up to 4 hours for maximum flavor.

13

- 1 teaspoon paprika
- 1 teaspoon ground cumin
- 1/2 teaspoon ground coriander
- 1/2 teaspoon ground turmeric
- Salt and pepper to taste
- Chopped fresh parsley

- Preheat the grill or grill pan to medium-high heat.
- Remove the chicken from the marinade and shake off any excess. Discard the remaining marinade.
- Grill the chicken breasts for 6-8 minutes per side, or until they are cooked through and reach an internal temperature of 165°F (75°C). Cooking time may vary depending on the thickness of the chicken breasts.
- Once cooked, remove the chicken from the grill and let it rest for a few minutes before serving.

Nutritional information

- Calories:150kcal
- Fat: 10g
- Carbohydrates: 5g
- Protein: 15g
- Fiber: 3g
- Sodium: 300mg

Instant Pot Stuffed Cinnamon Walnut Apples

Prep time: 10 minutes
Cook time: 10 minutes
Servings: 6

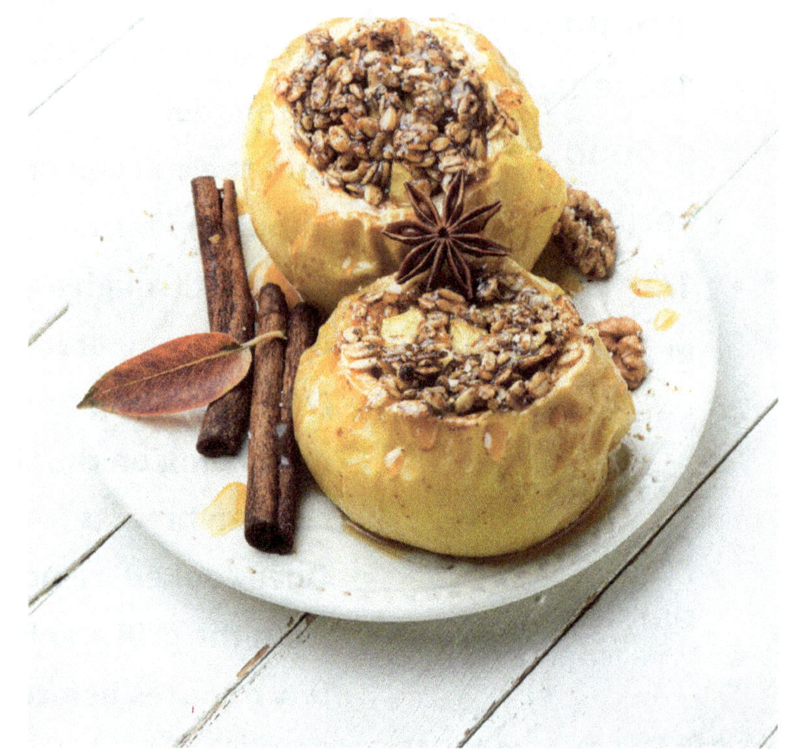

Ingredients:

- 4 large apples
- 1/2 cup chopped walnuts
- 1/4 cup raisins or dried cranberries
- 2 tablespoons brown sugar

Procedure:

- Wash the apples and carefully core them, removing the seeds and creating a hollow cavity in the center. You can use an apple corer or a small knife to do this. Be sure not to cut all the way through the bottom of the apples.
- In a mixing bowl, combine the chopped walnuts, raisins or dried cranberries, brown sugar or maple syrup, ground cinnamon, and ground nutmeg. Mix well to create the stuffing mixture.

- **1 teaspoon ground cinnamon**
- **1/4 teaspoon ground nutmeg**
- **1 cup apple juice or water.**

- Stuff each cored apple with the walnut and raisin mixture, pressing it down gently to fill the entire hollow cavity.
- Pour the apple juice or water into the inner pot of your Instant Pot.
- Place a trivet or steamer basket in the Instant Pot, then arrange the stuffed apples on top of the trivet or basket.
- Close the lid of the Instant Pot and set the valve to the sealing position. Select the "Manual" or "Pressure Cook" setting and set the cooking time to 5 minutes at high pressure.
- Once the cooking cycle is complete, allow the pressure to naturally release for 5 minutes, then carefully perform a quick release to release any remaining pressure.
- Carefully remove the stuffed apples from the Instant Pot using tongs or a slotted spoon, as they will be hot.
- Serve the Instant Pot Stuffed Cinnamon Walnut Apples warm.

Nutritional information

- **Calories: 150kcal**
- **Fat: 5g**
- **Carbohydrates: 25g**
- **Protein: 5g**
- **Fiber: 6g**
- **Sugar: 25g**
- **Sodium: 100mg**

Instant Pot Fish Taco Bowls

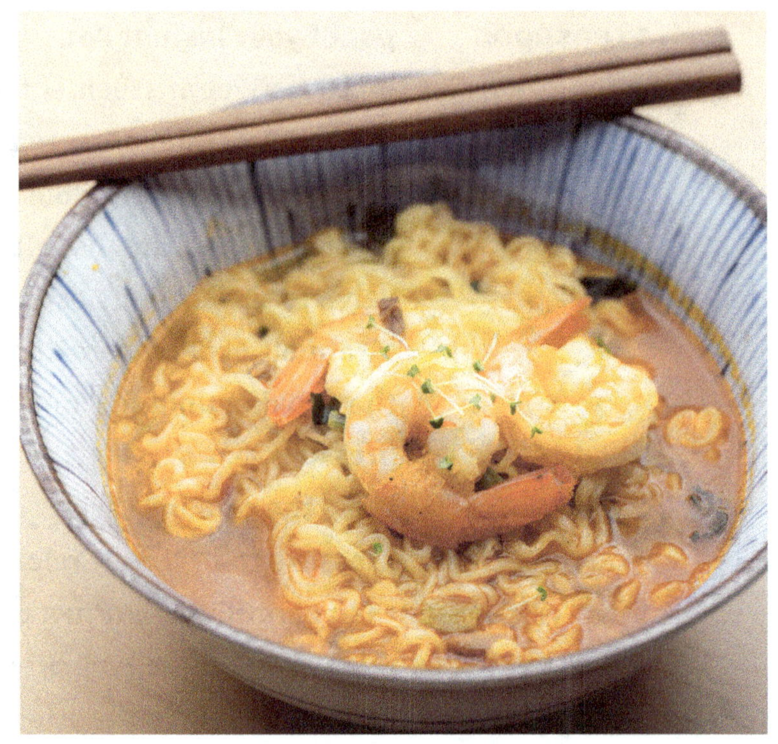

Prep time: 3 minutes
Cook time: 3 minutes

Servings: 4

Ingredients:

- 1 pound white fish fillets (such as tilapia or cod), cut into chunks
- 1 tablespoon olive oil
- 1 small onion, diced
- 1 bell pepper, diced
- 1 jalapeño pepper, seeded and minced.

Procedure:

- Set your Instant Pot to "Sauté" mode and heat the olive oil. Add the diced onion, bell pepper, jalapeño pepper, and minced garlic. Sauté for 2-3 minutes, or until the vegetables are softened.

- Add the taco seasoning to the vegetables and stir to coat.

- Add the white fish chunks to the Instant Pot, stirring gently to combine with the vegetables.

17

- 2 cloves garlic, minced
- 1 tablespoon taco seasoning
- 1 cup corn kernels (fresh, frozen, or canned)
- 1 can (15 ounces) black beans, drained and rinsed
- 1 cup rice, rinsed
- 1 cup chicken or vegetable broth.

- Add the corn kernels, black beans, rinsed rice, and chicken or vegetable broth to the Instant Pot. Season with salt and pepper to taste.
- Close the lid of the Instant Pot and set the valve to the sealing position. Select the "Manual" or "Pressure Cook" setting and set the cooking time to 3 minutes at high pressure.
- Once the cooking cycle is complete, perform a quick release to release the pressure.
- Carefully open the lid of the Instant Pot and fluff the contents of the pot with a fork.
- Serve the Instant Pot Fish Taco Bowls hot, garnished with chopped fresh cilantro, diced avocado, shredded cheese, salsa, sour cream, and lime wedges.

Nutritional Information

- Calories: 400 kcal
- Fat: 10g
- Carbohydrates: 30g
- Protein: 30g
- Fiber: 8g
- Sodium: 600mg

Instant Pot Sweet Potatoes Nachos

Prep time: 10 minutes
Cook time: 20 minutes
Servings: 4

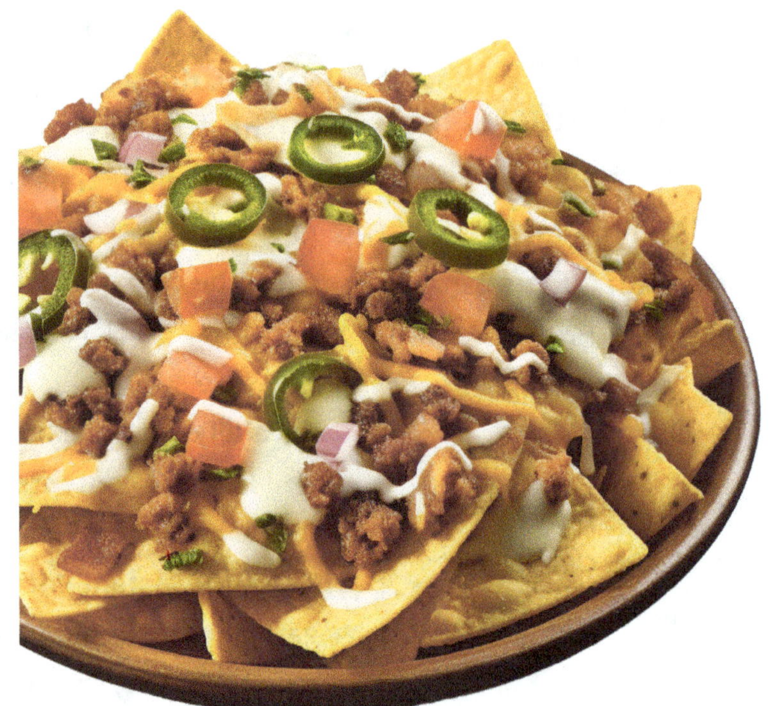

Ingredients:

- 2 large sweet potatoes, thinly sliced into rounds
- 1 tablespoon olive oil
- 1 teaspoon chili powder
- 1/2 teaspoon cumin
- 1/2 teaspoon paprika
- Salt and pepper to taste

Procedure:

- In a mixing bowl, toss the thinly sliced sweet potatoes with olive oil, chili powder, cumin, paprika, salt, and pepper until evenly coated.
- Place the seasoned sweet potato slices in the bottom of the Instant Pot, arranging them in a single layer.
- Sprinkle shredded cheese over the sweet potato slices, followed by black beans, corn kernels, diced red onion, and diced jalapeño.

19

- **1 cup shredded cheese (cheddar, Monterey Jack, or a blend)**
- **1/2 cup black beans, drained and rinsed**
- **1/2 cup corn kernels (fresh, frozen, or canned)**
- **1/4 cup diced red onion**
- **1/4 cup diced jalapeño**
- **1/4 cup chopped fresh cilantro.**

- **Close the lid of the Instant Pot and set the valve to the sealing position. Select the "Manual" or "Pressure Cook" setting and set the cooking time to 10 minutes at high pressure.**
- **Once the cooking cycle is complete, perform a quick release to release the pressure.**
- **Carefully open the lid of the Instant Pot and transfer the sweet potato nachos to a serving platter or individual plates.**
- **Garnish the sweet potato nachos with chopped fresh cilantro and any desired toppings, such as diced avocado, sliced black olives, sour cream, salsa, or guacamole.**
- **Serve the Instant Pot Sweet Potato Nachos hot and enjoy immediately.**

Nutritional Information

- **Calories: 175kcal**
- **Total Fat: 1g**
- **Cholesterol: 4mg**
- **Sodium: 227 mg**
- **Carbohydrates: 31g**
- **Fiber: 6g**
- **Sugars: 9g**
- **Protein: 10g**

Grilled Salmon Kebabs

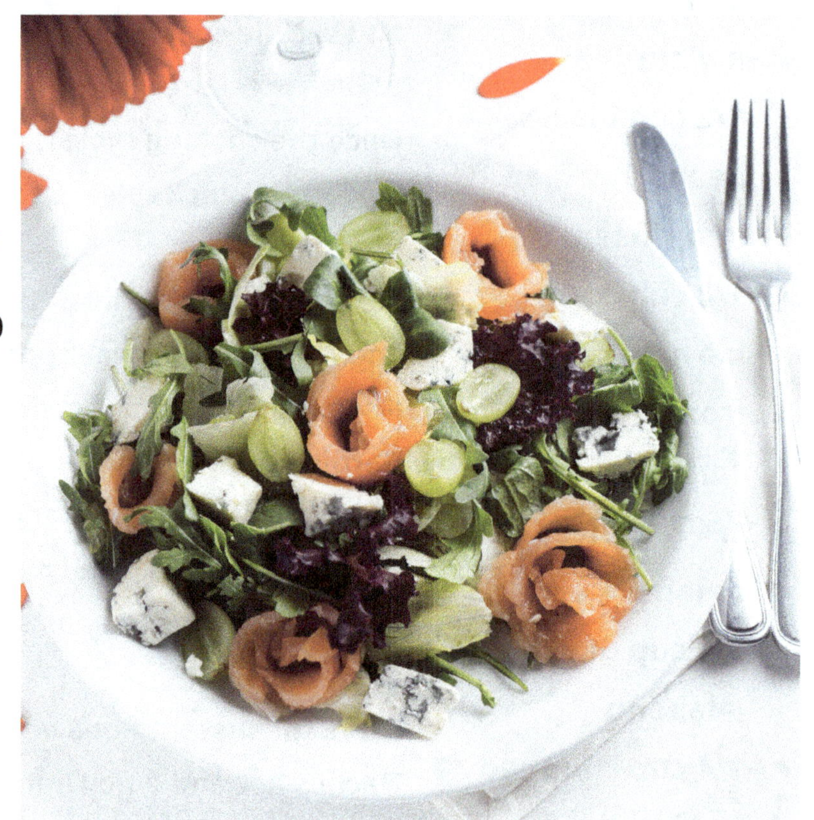

Prep time: 15 minutes
Cook time: 10 minutes
Servings: 4

Ingredients:

- 1 pound salmon fillets, skin removed and cut into 1-inch cubes
- 2 tablespoons olive oil
- 2 cloves garlic, minced.

Procedure:

- If using wooden skewers, soak them in water for at least 30 minutes to prevent burning.
- In a bowl, combine the olive oil, minced garlic, lemon juice, dried oregano, dried thyme, paprika, salt, and pepper. Mix well to create the marinade.
- Add the salmon cubes to the marinade, tossing to coat evenly. Allow the salmon to marinate in the refrigerator for at least 30 minutes, or up to 2 hours for more flavor.

21

- 1 tablespoon lemon juice
- 1 teaspoon dried oregano
- 1 teaspoon dried thyme
- 1/2 teaspoon paprika
- Salt and pepper to taste

- Preheat the grill to medium-high heat
- Thread the marinated salmon cubes onto skewers.
- Place the salmon kebabs on the preheated grill and cook for 3-4 minutes per side, or until the salmon is cooked through and flakes easily with a fork.
- Once cooked, remove the salmon kebabs from the grill and transfer them to a serving platter.
- Serve the grilled salmon kebabs hot.

Nutritional Information

- Calories: 267kcal
- Carbohydrates: 7g
- Protein: 35g
- Fat: 11g
- Cholesterol: 94 mg
- Sodium: 658 mg
- Fiber: 3g

Shoyu Ahi Tuna Poke

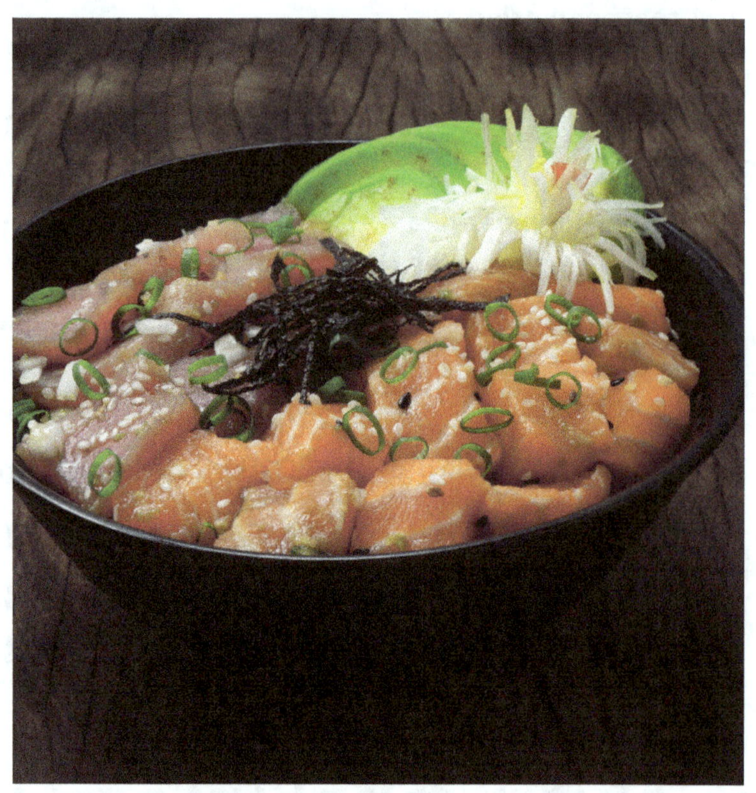

Prep time: 3 minutes
Cook time: 3 minutes
Servings: 4

Ingredients:

- 1 pound sushi-grade ahi tuna, cubed
- 2 tablespoons soy sauce
- 1 tablespoon sesame oil.

Procedure:

- In a mixing bowl, combine the cubed ahi tuna with soy sauce, sesame oil, rice vinegar, grated fresh ginger, and minced garlic. Gently toss to coat the tuna evenly in the marinade. Cover the bowl and refrigerate for at least 30 minutes to allow the flavors to meld.

- 1 tablespoon rice vinegar
- 1 teaspoon grated fresh ginger
- 1 teaspoon minced garlic
- 1 green onion, thinly sliced
- 1 tablespoon sesame seeds.

- While the tuna is marinating, prepare any optional toppings you plan to use.
- After the tuna has marinated, remove it from the refrigerator and add sliced green onions and sesame seeds. Gently toss to combine.
- Serve the shoyu ahi tuna poke in bowls, topped with your desired toppings such as sliced avocado, sliced cucumber, seaweed salad, edamame, sliced radishes, and sliced jalapeños.

Nutritional Information

- Calories: 166kcal
- Carbohydrates: 2.5g
- Protein: 28.5 g
- Fat: 4g
- Cholesterol: 44 mg
- Sodium: 512 mg
- Fiber: 0.5g
- Sugar: 0.6g

Chicken Enchilada Stuffed Zucchini Boats

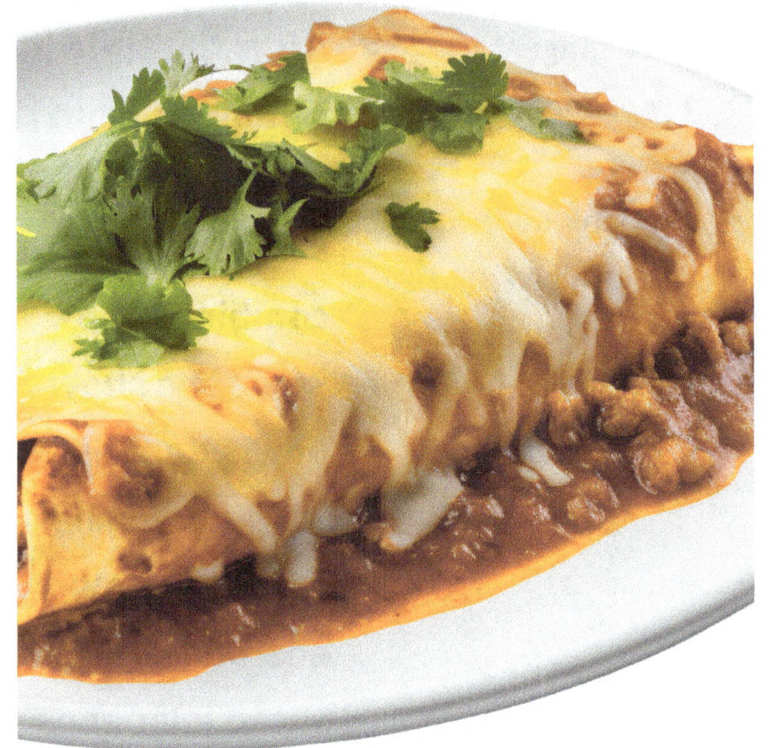

Prep time: 15 minutes
Cook time: 45 minutes
Servings: 4

Ingredients:

- 4 medium zucchini
- 2 cups cooked shredded chicken
- 1 cup enchilada sauce
- 1 cup shredded cheese

Procedure:

- For the enchilada sauce:
- In a medium saucepan, spray oil and sauté garlic.
- Add chipotle chiles, chili powder, cumin, chicken broth, tomato sauce, salt and pepper and bring to a boil.
- Reduce the heat to low and simmer for 5-10 minutes. Set aside until ready to use.

- 1/4 cup chopped fresh cilantro
- 1 teaspoon ground cumin
- 1/2 teaspoon chili powder
- 1/2 teaspoon garlic powder
- salt and pepper to taste.

- For the Zucchini Boats
- Preheat oven to 400°F.
- Cut zucchini in half lengthwise and using a small spoon or melon baller, scoop out flesh, leaving 1/4" thick.
- Chop the scooped out flesh of the zucchini in small pieces and set aside.
- In a large saute pan, heat oil and add onion, garlic and bell pepper.
- Cook on medium-low heat for about 2-3 minutes, until tender.i
- Add chopped zucchini and cilantro; season with salt and pepper and cook about 4 minutes.
- Add the cumin, oregano, chili powder, water, and tomato paste and cook a few more minutes, then add in chicken; mix and cook 3 more minutes.
- Place 1/4 cup of the enchilada sauce on the bottom of a large (or 2 small) baking dish, and place zucchini halves cut side up.
- Using a spoon, fill each hollowed zucchini with 1/3 cup chicken mixture, pressing firmly.
- Top each with 2 tablespoons of enchilada sauce, and 1 1/2 tablespoons each of shredded cheese.
- Cover with foil and bake 35 minutes until cheese is melted and zucchini is tender.
- Top with scallions and cilantro for garnish and serve with Greek yogurt or sour cream.

Nutritional Information

- Calories: 232 kcal
- Carbohydrates: 22g
- Protein: 24g
- Fat: 7g
- Cholesterol: 44 mg
- Sodium: 820 mg
- Fiber: 6g
- Sugar: 9g

Banana Souffle

Prep time: 5 minutes
Cook time: 3 minutes
Servings: 1

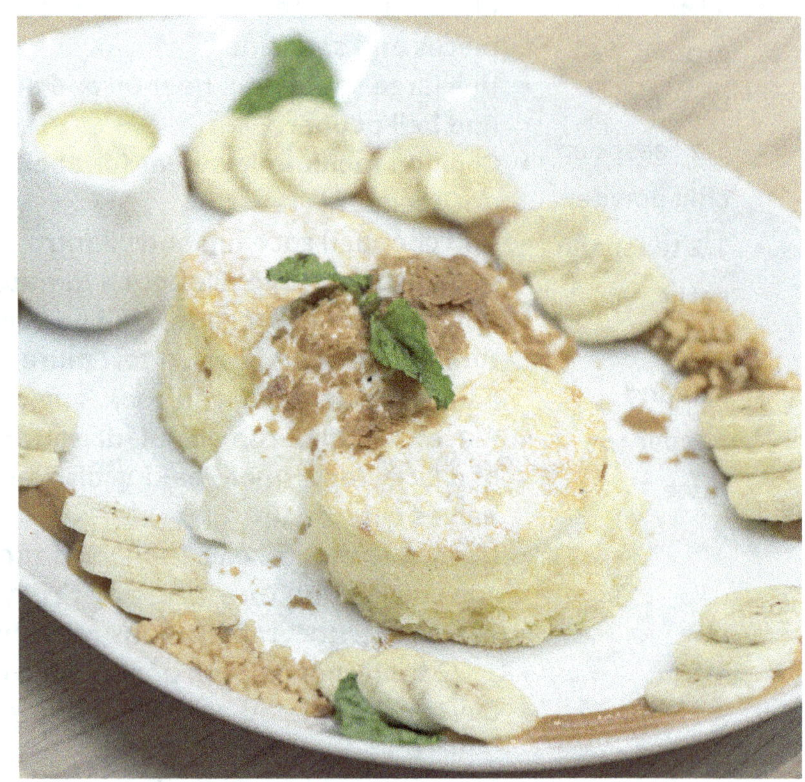

Ingredients:

- 2 ripe bananas
- 3 large eggs, separated
- 1/4 cup granulated sugar
- 1/4 teaspoon vanilla extract
- Pinch of salt

Procedure:

- Preheat your oven to 375°F (190°C). Grease four ramekins or oven-safe dishes with butter or cooking spray.
- Peel the ripe bananas and mash them in a mixing bowl until smooth.
- In a separate mixing bowl, beat the egg yolks with granulated sugar until pale and creamy. Stir in the mashed bananas and vanilla extract until well combined.

27

- In another clean mixing bowl, beat the egg whites with a pinch of salt until stiff peaks form.
- Gently fold the beaten egg whites into the banana mixture, being careful not to deflate the egg whites.
- Divide the soufflé mixture evenly among the prepared ramekins, filling them about three-quarters full.
- Place the ramekins on a baking sheet and transfer them to the preheated oven.
- Bake the banana soufflés for 12-15 minutes, or until they are puffed up and golden brown on top.
- Remove the soufflés from the oven and serve immediately, dusted with powdered sugar and topped with sliced bananas, whipped cream, or vanilla ice cream.

Nutritional Information

- Calories: 336kcal
- Carbohydrates: 55g
- Protein: 14g
- Fat: 9g
- Cholesterol: 327mg
- Sodium: 127mg
- Potassium: 966mg
- Fiber: 6g
- Sugar: 29g
- Vitamin A: 626IU
- Vitamin C: 21mg
- Calcium: 61mg
- Iron: 2mg

Egg roll in a bowl

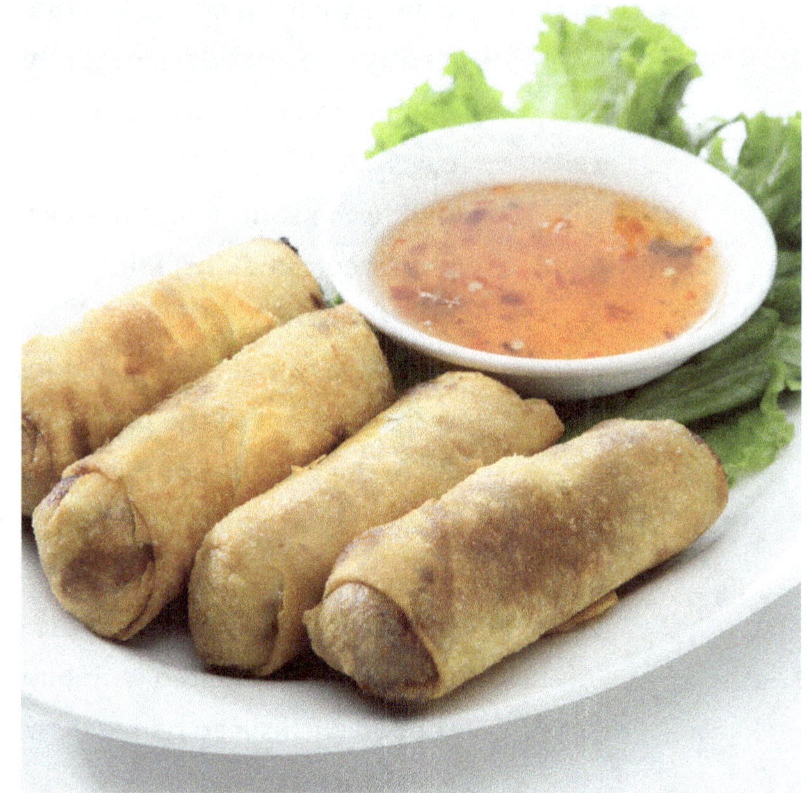

Prep time: 10 minutes
Cook time: 15 minutes

Servings: 6

Ingredients:

- 1 pound ground pork or chicken
- 1 tablespoon sesame oil
- 1 small onion, finely chopped
- 3 cloves garlic, minced
- 1 tablespoon freshly grated ginger.

Procedure:

- Heat the sesame oil in a large skillet or wok over medium-high heat.
- Add the ground pork or chicken to the skillet and cook, breaking it apart with a spatula, until browned and cooked through.
- Add the chopped onion, minced garlic, and grated ginger to the skillet. Cook, stirring frequently, for 2-3 minutes, or until the onion is translucent and fragrant.

29

- 1/4 cup soy sauce
- 1 tablespoon rice vinegar
- 1 tablespoon Sriracha sauce (adjust to taste)
- 1 small head cabbage, thinly sliced
- 2 medium carrots, julienned or grated
- 4 green onions, thinly sliced

- In a small bowl, whisk together the soy sauce, rice vinegar, and Sriracha sauce.
- Pour the sauce mixture into the skillet with the cooked meat and vegetables. Stir to combine.
- Add the thinly sliced cabbage and julienned or grated carrots to the skillet. Cook, stirring frequently, for 5-6 minutes, or until the cabbage is wilted and the carrots are tender-crisp.
- Stir in the sliced green onions and cook for an additional 1-2 minutes.
- Taste the egg roll in a bowl and adjust the seasoning if needed, adding more soy sauce or Sriracha sauce
- Remove the skillet from the heat and transfer the egg roll in a bowl to serving plates.
- Garnish the egg roll in a bowl with sesame seeds, sliced green onions, and sliced red chili peppers.

Nutritional Information

- Calories: 159kcal
- Carbohydrates: 15g
- Protein: 21g
- Fat: 2g
- Cholesterol: 48mg
- Sodium: 694mg
- Potassium: 740mg
- Fiber: 5g
- Sugar: 7g
- Vitamin A: 171IU
- Vitamin C: 59mg
- Calcium: 71mg
- Iron: 2mg

Skinny strawberry-Banana Bread

Prep time: 20 minutes
Cook time: 1 hr
Servings: 1

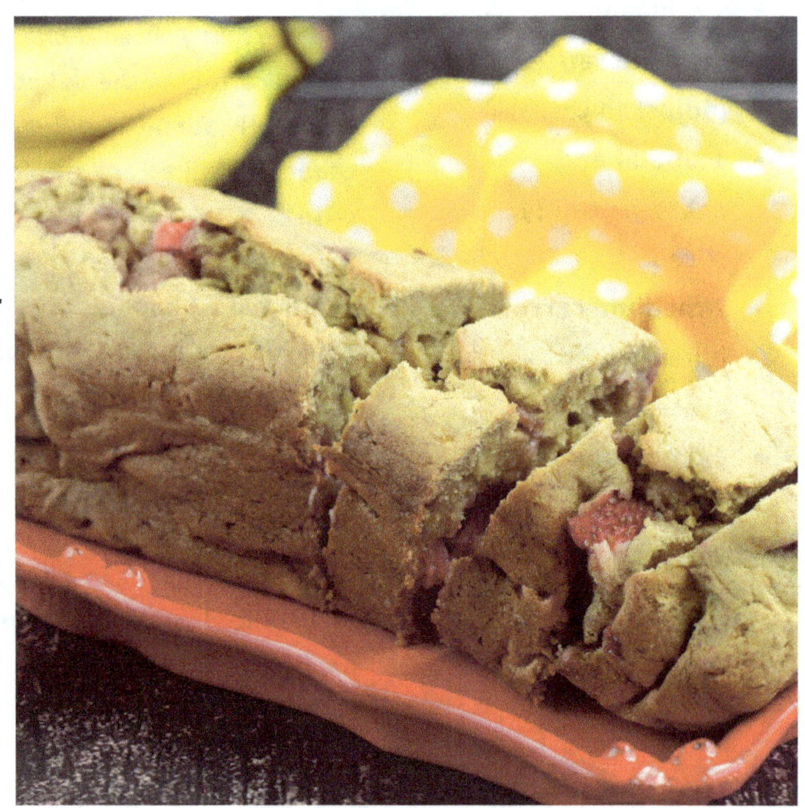

Ingredients:

- 1 cup mashed ripe bananas (about 2 medium bananas)
- 1/2 cup plain Greek yogurt
- 1/4 cup honey or maple syrup
- 1/4 cup unsweetened applesauce
- 2 eggs
- 1 teaspoon vanilla extract.

Procedure:

- Preheat your oven to 350°F (175°C). Grease a 9x5-inch loaf pan with cooking spray or line it with parchment paper.
- In a large mixing bowl, combine mashed bananas, Greek yogurt, honey or maple syrup, unsweetened applesauce, eggs, and vanilla extract. Mix until smooth.

- **1 and 1/2 cups whole wheat flour or all-purpose flour**
- **1 teaspoon baking soda**
- **1/2 teaspoon baking powder**
- **1/2 teaspoon cinnamon**
- **1/4 teaspoon salt**
- **1 cup chopped strawberries**

- In a separate bowl, whisk together flour, baking soda, baking powder, cinnamon, and salt.
- Gradually add dry ingredients to wet ingredients, stirring until just combined. Do not overmix.
- Gently fold in chopped strawberries until evenly distributed throughout the batter
- Pour the batter into the prepared loaf pan and spread it out evenly.
- Bake for 50-60 minutes, or until a toothpick inserted into the center comes out clean.
- Allow the bread to cool in the pan for 10 minutes before transferring to a wire rack to cool completely.

Nutritional Information

- **Calories: 87kcal**
- **Carbohydrates: 15g**
- **Protein: 1g**
- **Fat: 3g**
- **Saturated Fat: 2g**
- **Sodium: 55mg**
- **Fiber: 1g**
- **Sugar: 7g**

Crockpot Chicken Tortilla Soup

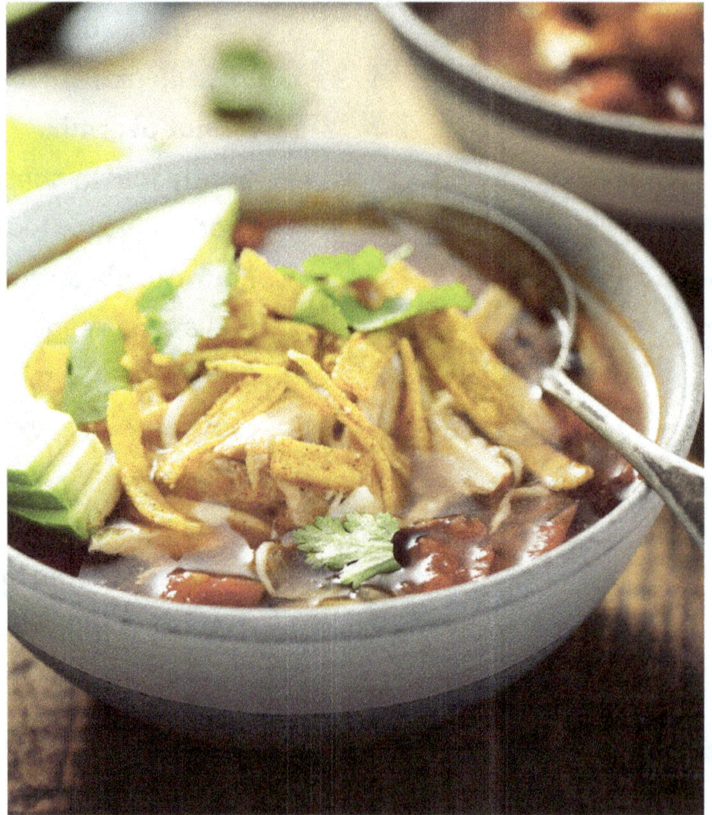

Prep time: 10 minutes
Cook time: 6 hours
Servings: 1

Ingredients:

- 1 pound boneless, skinless chicken breasts or thighs
- 1 can (14.5 ounces) diced tomatoes
- 1 can (15 ounces) black beans, drained and rinsed
- 1 can (15 ounces) corn kernels, drained

Procedure:

- Place the chicken breasts or thighs in the bottom of the crockpot.
- Add diced tomatoes, black beans, corn kernels, diced onion, diced bell pepper, minced garlic, and diced jalapeño pepper to the crockpot.
- Pour chicken broth over the ingredients in the crockpot.
- Sprinkle chili powder, ground cumin, paprika, salt, and pepper over the ingredients in the crockpot.

- 1 onion, diced
- 1 bell pepper, diced
- 2 cloves garlic, minced
- 1 jalapeño pepper, diced
- 4 cups chicken broth
- 1 tablespoon chili powder
- 1 teaspoon ground cumin
- 1 teaspoon paprika
- Salt and pepper to taste
- Juice of 1 lime
- Tortilla chips.

- Cover and cook on low heat for 6-8 hours or on high heat for 3-4 hours, or until the chicken is cooked through and tender.
- Once the chicken is cooked, remove it from the crockpot and shred it using two forks. Return the shredded chicken to the crockpot.
- Stir in the lime juice and adjust the seasoning if needed, adding more salt and pepper to taste.
- Serve the crockpot chicken tortilla soup hot, ladled into bowls and topped with crushed tortilla chips.
- Garnish with shredded cheese, diced avocado, sour cream, chopped cilantro, and lime wedges.

Nutritional Information

- Calories: 256kcal
- Carbohydrates: 31.3g
- Protein: 26g
- Fat: 3.4g
- Saturated Fat: 0.3g
- Cholesterol: 48mg
- Sodium: 532 mg
- Potassium: 841mg
- Fiber: 7.6g
- Sugar: 4.3g
- Calcium: 70mg
- Iron: 4.1mg

Slow Cooker Chicken Cacciatore

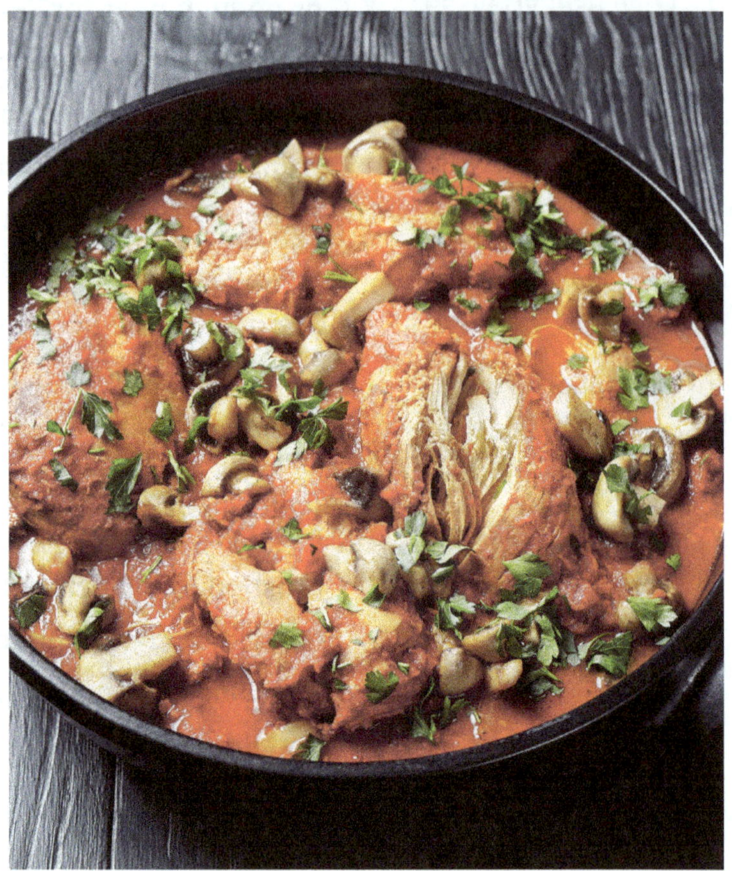

Prep time: 30 minutes
Cook time: 4 hours
Servings: 1

Ingredients:

- 4 bone-in, skin-on chicken thighs
- 4 bone-in, skin-on chicken drumsticks
- Salt and pepper to taste
- 2 tablespoons olive oil
- 1 onion, thinly sliced
- 1 bell pepper, thinly sliced
- 2 cloves garlic, minced

Procedure:

- Season the chicken thighs and drumsticks generously with salt and pepper.
- Heat olive oil in a large skillet over medium-high heat. Add the chicken pieces and brown them on all sides, about 3-4 minutes per side. Transfer the browned chicken to the slow cooker.
- In the same skillet, add sliced onion and bell pepper. Cook until softened, about 3-4 minutes. Add minced garlic and cook for an additional 1 minute.
- Add diced tomatoes, tomato paste, chicken broth, dried oregano, dried basil, dried thyme, dried rosemary, and red pepper flakes to the skillet. Stir to combine and bring the mixture to a simmer.

35

- 1 can (14.5 ounces) diced tomatoes
- 1 can (6 ounces) tomato paste
- 1/2 cup chicken broth
- 1 teaspoon dried oregano
- 1 teaspoon dried basil
- 1/2 teaspoon dried thyme
- 1/2 teaspoon dried rosemary
- 1/2 teaspoon red pepper flakes (optional, for added heat)
- 1/4 cup chopped fresh parsley, for garnish
- Cooked pasta or rice for serving.

- Pour the tomato mixture over the chicken in the slow cooker.
- Cover and cook on low heat for 6-8 hours or on high heat for 3-4 hours, or until the chicken is cooked through and tender.
- Once the chicken is cooked, remove it from the slow cooker and transfer it to a serving platter.
- Skim any excess fat from the surface of the sauce in the slow cooker. Taste the sauce and adjust the seasoning
- Serve the chicken cacciatore hot, garnished with chopped fresh parsley, and accompanied by cooked pasta or rice.

Nutritional Information

- Calories: 311kcal
- Carbohydrates: 10g
- Protein: 21g
- Fat: 20g
- Cholesterol: 118mg
- Sodium: 444mg
- Potassium: 630mg
- Fiber: 2g
- Sugar: 5g
- Vitamin A: 610IU
- Vitamin C: 26.7mg
- Calcium: 49mg
- Iron: 2.3mg

Arizona Burrito Bowls

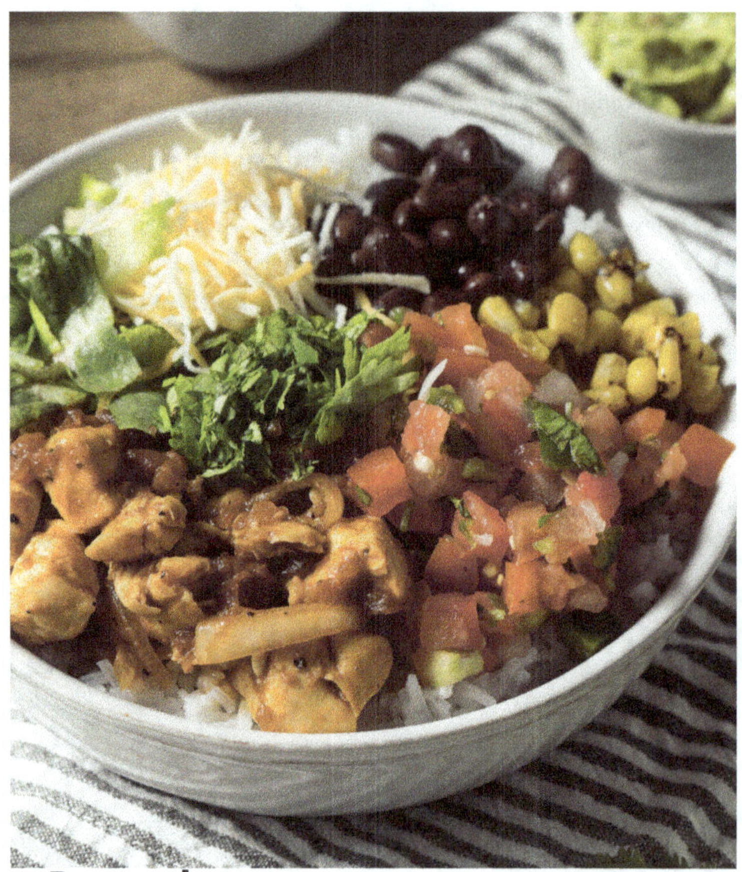

Ingredients:

- 1 pound ground beef or turkey
- 1 tablespoon olive oil
- 1 onion, diced
- 2 cloves garlic, minced
- 1 bell pepper, diced
- 1 cup corn kernels (fresh, frozen, or canned).

Procedure:

- Heat olive oil in a large skillet over medium-high heat. Add diced onion and cook until softened, about 3-4 minutes.
- Add ground beef or turkey to the skillet and cook until browned, breaking it apart with a spatula as it cooks.
- Stir in minced garlic and diced bell pepper. Cook for an additional 2-3 minutes.
- Add corn kernels, black beans, diced tomatoes with green chilies, chili powder, ground cumin, paprika, salt, and pepper to the skillet. Stir to combine.

37

- 1 can (15 ounces) black beans, drained and rinsed
- 1 can (10 ounces) diced tomatoes with green chilies
- 1 teaspoon chili powder
- 1/2 teaspoon ground cumin
- 1/2 teaspoon paprika
- Salt and pepper to taste
- Cooked rice for serving.

- Reduce the heat to medium-low and let the mixture simmer for 10-15 minutes, stirring occasionally, to allow the flavors to meld and the sauce to thicken.
- While the mixture is simmering, prepare cooked rice according to package instructions.
- Once the burrito bowl mixture is ready, serve it hot over cooked rice.
- Garnish the Arizona burrito bowls with shredded cheese, diced avocado, sliced jalapeños, chopped cilantro, sour cream, and salsa.

Nutritional Information

- Calories: 500kcal
- Fat: 15g
- Carbohydrates: 50g
- Protein: About 25g
- Fiber: 10g
- Sodium: 700mg

Baked Salmon With Fresh Herbs

Prep time: 5 minutes
Cook time: 25 minutes

Servings: 6

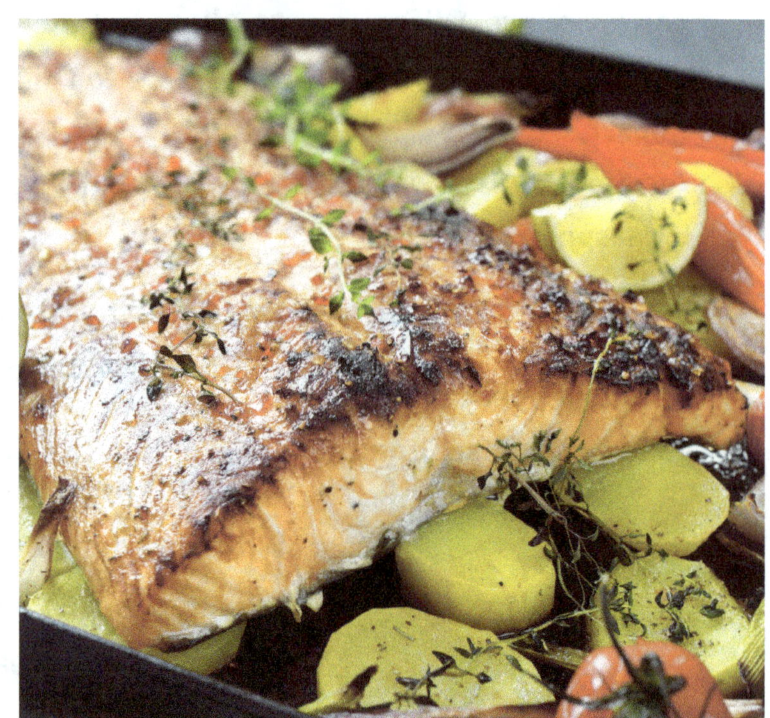

Ingredients:

- 4 salmon fillets, skin-on or skinless
- 2 tablespoons olive oil
- 2 cloves garlic, minced
- 2 tablespoons fresh lemon juice
- 2 tablespoons chopped fresh parsley.

Procedure:

- Preheat your oven to 375°F (190°C). Line a baking sheet with parchment paper or aluminum foil for easy cleanup.
- In a small bowl, mix together olive oil, minced garlic, fresh lemon juice, chopped parsley, chopped dill, and chopped chives to create the herb marinade.
- Place the salmon fillets on the prepared baking sheet. Season both sides of the salmon fillets with salt and pepper.
- Spoon the herb marinade over the salmon fillets, spreading it evenly to coat the surface of each fillet.

- 1 tablespoon chopped fresh dill
- 1 tablespoon chopped fresh chives
- Salt and pepper to taste
- Lemon slices for garnish.

- If using skin-on salmon, you can make a few shallow cuts on the skin side of the fillets to help the marinade penetrate.
- Let the salmon marinate for 10-15 minutes to allow the flavors to infuse.
- Once marinated, transfer the baking sheet to the preheated oven and bake the salmon for 12-15 minutes, or until the fish is cooked through and flakes easily with a fork. The cooking time may vary depending on the thickness of the salmon fillets.
- Once cooked, remove the salmon from the oven and let it rest for a few minutes before serving.
- Garnish the baked salmon with lemon slices, and serve hot.

Nutritional Information

- Calories: 233kcal
- Carbohydrates: 2g
- Protein: 30.5g
- Fat: 11g
- Saturated Fat: 1.5g
- Cholesterol: 83mg
- Sodium: 160mg
- Fiber: 1g

Spicy Popcorn

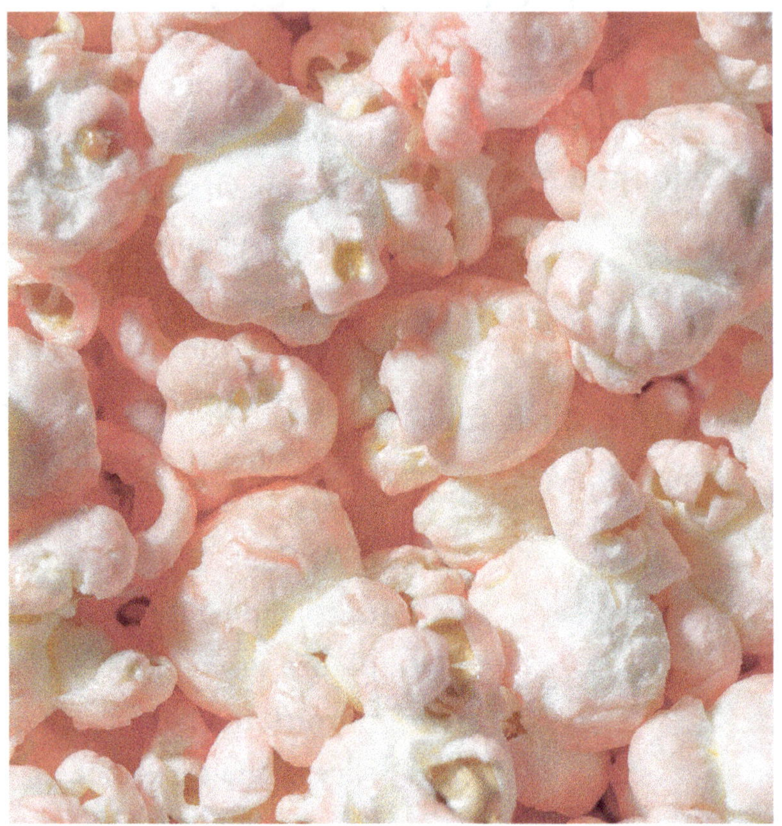

**Prep time: 5 minutes
Cook time: 10 minutes
Servings: 4**

Ingredients:

- 1/2 cup popcorn kernels
- 2 tablespoons vegetable oil or coconut oil
- 2 tablespoons unsalted butter, melted.

Procedure:

- Heat the vegetable oil or coconut oil in a large pot with a tight-fitting lid over medium-high heat.
- Add the popcorn kernels to the pot and cover with the lid. Shake the pot occasionally to ensure even heating and to prevent the kernels from burning.
- Once the popping slows down, remove the pot from the heat and let it sit for a few seconds to allow any remaining kernels to pop.

- 1 teaspoon chili powder
- 1/2 teaspoon paprika
- 1/4 teaspoon cayenne pepper
- Salt to taste.

- In a small bowl, mix together the melted butter, chili powder, paprika, cayenne pepper, and salt.
- Transfer the popped popcorn to a large bowl. Drizzle the spicy butter mixture over the popcorn and toss to coat evenly.
- Taste and adjust the seasoning if needed, adding more salt or cayenne pepper for extra spice.
- Serve the spicy popcorn immediately as a delicious snack or movie night treat.

Nutritional Information

- Calories: 150kcal
- Fat: 5g
- Carbohydrates: 10g
- Protein: 2g
- Fiber: 3g
- Sodium: 200mg

Veggie Frittata Spices

Prep time: 20 minutes
Cook time: 30 minutes
Servings: 4

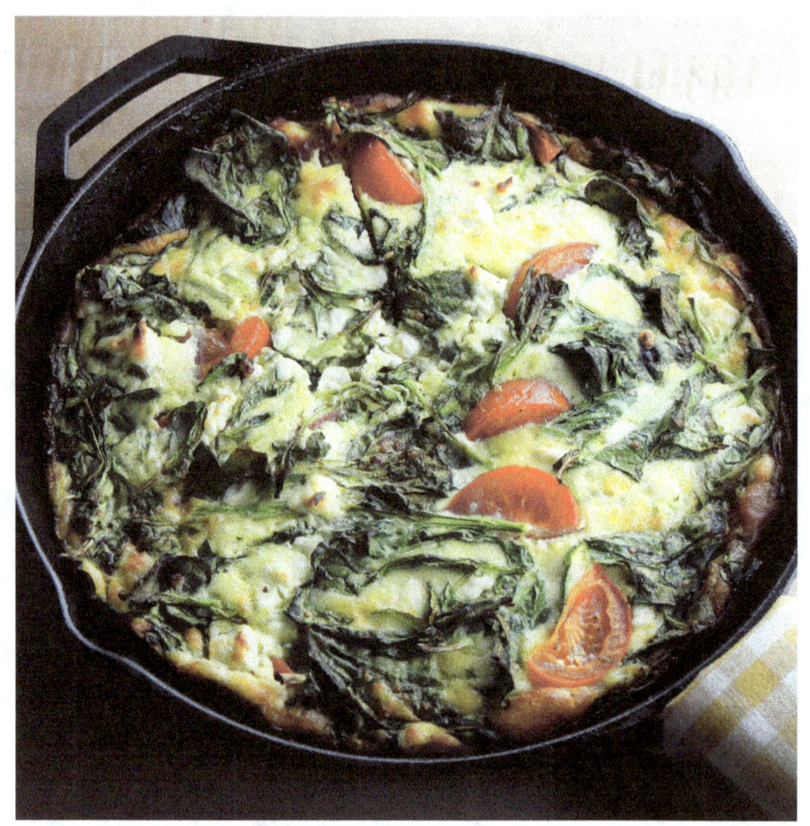

Ingredients:

- 8 large eggs
- 1/4 cup milk
- 1 cup chopped vegetables
- 1/2 cup shredded cheese.

Procedure:

- Preheat your oven to 350°F (175°C).
- In a large mixing bowl, crack the eggs and whisk them together with the milk until well combined. Season with salt and pepper to taste.
- Heat olive oil or butter in a skillet over medium heat. Add the chopped vegetables and sauté until they are softened, about 5-7 minutes.
- Spread the sautéed vegetables evenly in the skillet and pour the egg mixture over the top.

43

- 2 tablespoons olive oil or butter
- Salt and pepper to taste
- Fresh herbs.

- Sprinkle shredded cheese over the egg and vegetable mixture.
- Cook the frittata on the stovetop for 3-4 minutes, until the edges start to set.
- Transfer the skillet to the preheated oven and bake for 15-20 minutes, or until the frittata is set in the center and the top is golden brown.
- Once cooked, remove the frittata from the oven and let it cool for a few minutes.
- Slice the frittata into wedges or squares and garnish with fresh herbs if desired.
- Serve the veggie frittata slices warm or at room temperature.

Nutritional Information

- Calories: 150kcal
- Fat: 5g
- Carbohydrates: 10g
- Protein: 5g
- Fiber: 2g
- Sodium: 250mg

Air Fryer Ranch Turkey Burgers

Prep time: 5 minutes
Cook time: 30 minutes
Servings: 4

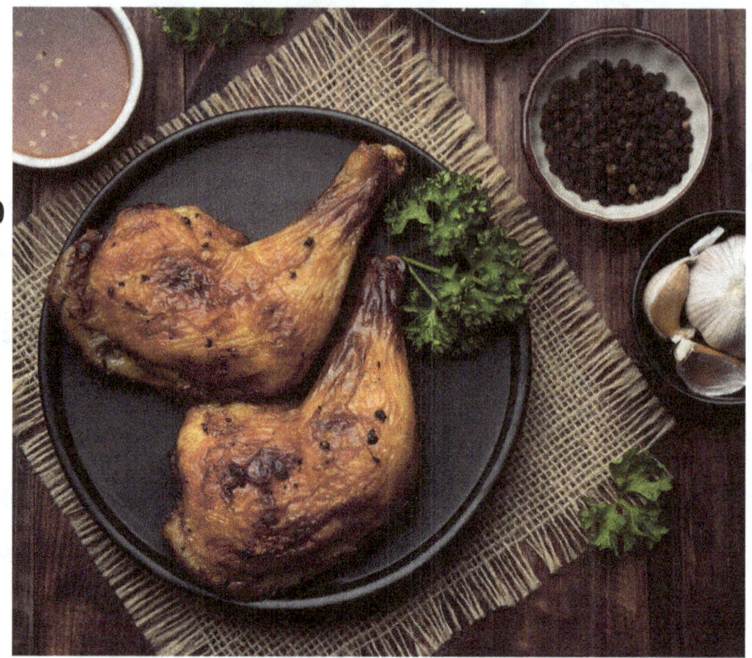

Ingredients:

- 1 pound ground turkey
- 1/4 cup breadcrumbs
- 2 tablespoons ranch seasoning mix
- 1/4 cup grated Parmesan cheese.

Procedure:

- In a mixing bowl, combine the ground turkey, breadcrumbs, ranch seasoning mix, grated Parmesan cheese, egg, salt, and pepper. Mix until well combined.
- Divide the turkey mixture into equal portions and shape them into burger patties.
- Preheat your air fryer to 375°F (190°C) for about 3-5 minutes.
- Place the turkey burger patties in the air fryer basket, making sure they are not overcrowded. You may need to cook them in batches depending on the size of your air fryer.

- **1 egg**
- **Salt and pepper to taste**
- **Burger buns**
- **Lettuce, tomato, onions.**

- Cook the turkey burgers in the air fryer for 12-15 minutes, flipping halfway through, or until they are cooked through and reach an internal temperature of 165°F (74°C).
- Once cooked
- Remove the turkey burgers from the air fryer and let them rest for a few minutes.
- While the burgers are resting, toast the burger buns in the air fryer for a couple of minutes.
- Assemble the turkey burgers by placing the cooked patties on the toasted buns and topping them with lettuce, tomato, onion, and any other toppings of your choice.

Nutritional Information

- Calories: 232kcal
- Carbohydrates: 7g
- Protein: 23g
- Fat: 12g
- Cholesterol: 95mg
- Sodium: 781mg
- Potassium: 278mg
- Fiber: 1g
- Sugar: 1g
- Vitamin A: 136IU
- Vitamin C: 1mg
- Calcium: 90mg
- Iron: 1mg

Apricot Chicken

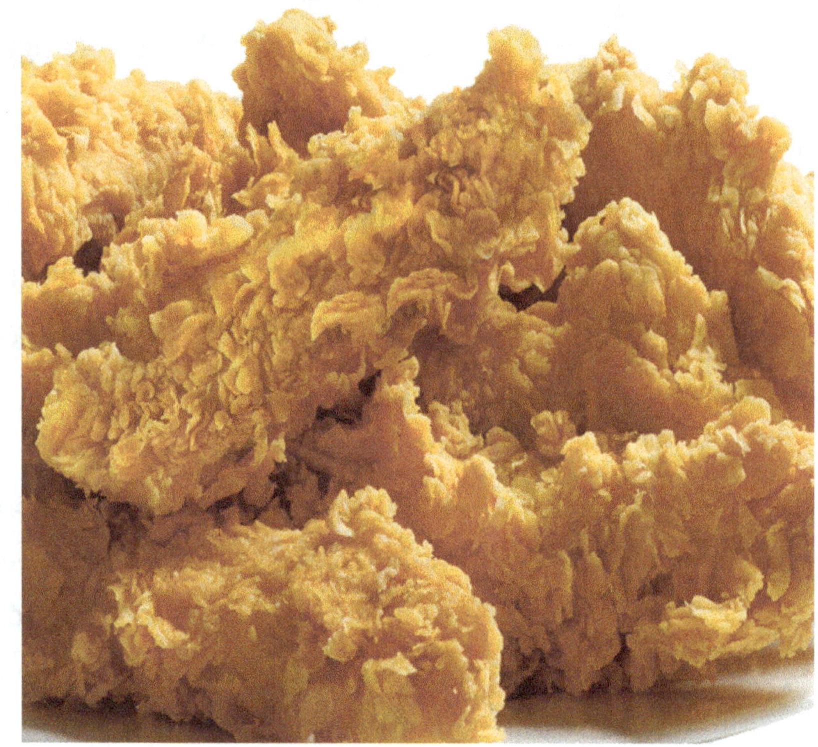

Prep time: 5 minutes
Cook time: 25 minutes
Servings: 4

Ingredients:

- 4 boneless, skinless chicken breasts
- Salt and pepper to taste
- 2 tablespoons olive oil
- 1 onion, diced
- 2 cloves garlic, minced
- 1 cup apricot preserves
- 1/4 cup soy sauce

Procedure:

- Preheat your oven to 375°F (190°C).
- Season the chicken breasts with salt and pepper on both sides.
- Heat olive oil in a large oven-safe skillet over medium-high heat. Add the chicken breasts and cook for 3-4 minutes on each side, or until they are browned. Remove the chicken from the skillet and set aside.
- In the same skillet, add diced onion and minced garlic. Cook until the onion is softened and translucent, about 3-4 minutes.

47

- 2 tablespoons Dijon mustard
- 1 tablespoon apple cider vinegar
- 1 teaspoon dried thyme
- 1/2 teaspoon dried rosemary
- 1/4 teaspoon red pepper flakes
- Chopped fresh parsley for garnish.

- Stir in apricot preserves, soy sauce, Dijon mustard, apple cider vinegar, dried thyme, dried rosemary, and red pepper flakes. Mix until well combined and heated through.
- Return the browned chicken breasts to the skillet, spooning the apricot mixture over the top.
- Transfer the skillet to the preheated oven and bake for 20-25 minutes, or until the chicken is cooked through and reaches an internal temperature of 165°F (74°C).
- Once cooked, remove the skillet from the oven and let it rest for a few minutes.
- Serve the apricot chicken hot, garnished with chopped fresh parsley.

Nutritional Information

- Calories: 300kcal
- Carbohydrates: 9g
- Protein: 49g
- Fat: 6g
- Cholesterol: 145mg
- Sodium: 187mg
- Potassium: 1001mg
- Fiber: 1g | Sugar: 6g
- Vitamin A: 803IU
- Vitamin C: 17mg
- Calcium: 22mg
- Iron: 1mg

Apple Cinnamon Wonder Whip

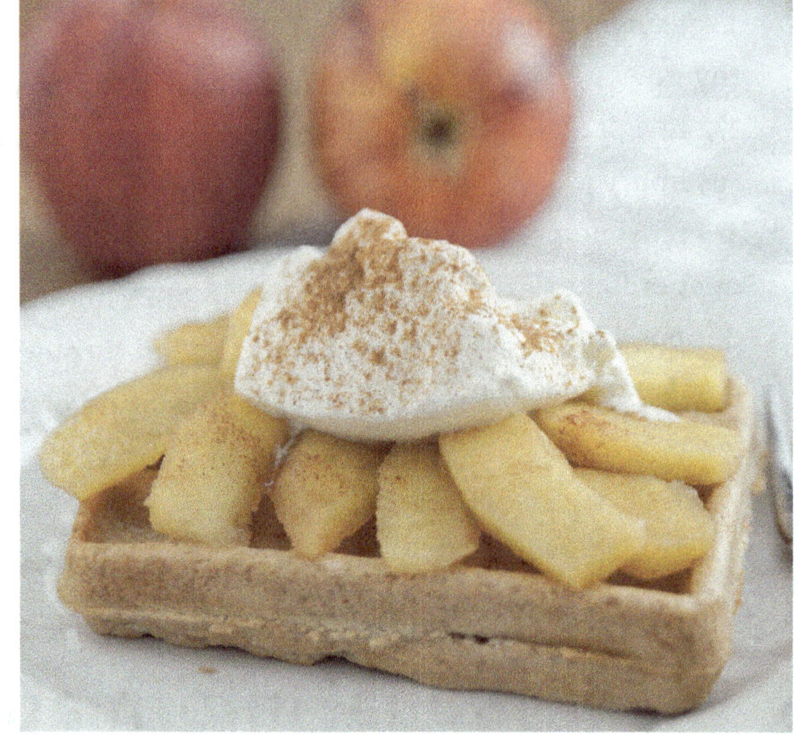

Prep time: 5 minutes
Cook time: 5 minutes
Servings: 1

Ingredients:

- 1/2 apple diced
- 3/4 cup Greek yogurt
- 1 tsp cinnamon.

Procedure:

- Whip together all ingredients using a fork, whisk, blender, or mixer.

Nutritional Information

- Calories: 170kcal
- Carbohydrates: 21g
- Protein: 20g
- Fat: 0g
- Cholesterol: 10mg
- Sodium: 73mg
- Potassium: 379mg
- Fiber: 3g
- Sugar: 15g
- Vitamin C: 4.2mg
- Calcium: 240mg

Chicken Gyro Bowls With Homemade Tzatziki

Prep time: 10 minutes
Cook time: 15 minutes
Servings: 6

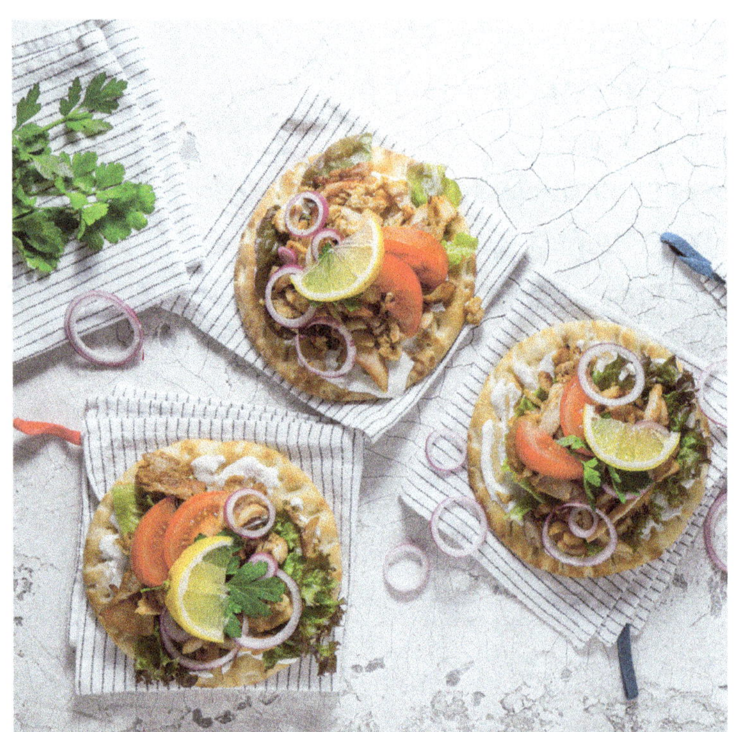

Ingredients:

- **Chicken Gyro Bowls**
- **1 spaghetti squash about 3 lbs**
- **1 – 1.5 lbs chicken thighs about 6 thighs**
- **2 tsp olive oil**
- **1/2 tbsp garlic powder**
- **1 tsp oregano dried**
- **1 tsp rosemary dried**
- **1/2 tsp pepper**

Procedure:

- Instant pot
- Cut the spaghetti squash in half and scoop out the seeds in the middle.
- In a large bowl, mix together all the ingredients for the chicken. The chicken should be completely covered in olive oil and seasoning.
- Turn the Instant Pot to sauté. When the Instant Pot is hot, sauté the chicken on each side for 2-3 minutes. Remove the chicken and set aside.
- Add 1 cup of water the Instant Pot insert and place the trivet on the bottom. Arrange the spaghetti squash on top of the trivet and place the chicken around the spaghetti squash.
- Close the lid and cook on high pressure using the manual setting for 10 minutes. Let the pressure release naturally.
- Remove the chicken and spaghetti squash. Chop the chicken while the spaghetti squash cool. When the spaghetti squash is cool enough to handle, use a fork to school out the "noodles." They should come right out.
- Assemble your bowls by placing the spaghetti squash on the bottom and topping it with diced chicken, cucumbers, tomatoes, red onions, basil, and Tzatziki sauce.

- 1/2 cup basil fresh, chopped
- 1 onion red, chopped
- 1 cucumber sliced
- 1 cup cherry tomatoes sliced in half
- Homemade Tzatziki Sauce
- 3/4 cup Greek yogurt plain
- 1 cup cucumber peeled, seeded, and chopped
- 1 clove garlic minced
- 1 tsp pepper
- 2 tbsp dill fresh.

- Oven and Stove Top
- Preheat the oven to 400 degrees. Cut the spaghetti squash in half and scoop out the seed. Place the squash cut side down on a baking pan. Bake for 30-45 minutes. 1 spaghetti squash
- In a large bowl mix together all the ingredients for the chicken. The chicken should be completely covered in olive oil and seasoning.
- Heat a skillet on medium high heat on the stove. Brown the chicken on each side for 2-3 minutes, then reduce the heat to medium and finish cooking the chicken for another 10-12 minutes or until done. Remove the chicken the heat and dice.
- When the spaghetti squash is done cooking allow it to cool, then scoop out the noodles.
- Assemble your bowls by placing the spaghetti squash on the bottom and topping it with diced chicken, cucumbers, tomatoes, red onions, basil, and Tzatziki sauce.
-
- Slow cooker
- Cut the spaghetti squash in half and scoop out the seeds. Place the squash cut side down in the slow cooker.
- In a large bowl, mix together all the ingredients for the chicken. The chicken should be completely covered in olive oil and seasoning.
- Heat a skillet on medium high heat on the stove. Brown the chicken on each side for 2-3 minutes then transfer the chicken to slow cooker. Arrange the chicken around the spaghetti squash.
- Add 1/2 cup water the slow cooker then cover the slow cooker with the lid. Cook on low heat for 4-6 hour or high heat for 2-3 hours.
- Remove the spaghetti squash and let cool before scooping out the noodles. Chop the chicken and assemble the bowls by placing the spaghetti squash on the bottom and topping it with diced chicken, cucumbers, tomatoes, red onions, basil, and Tzatziki sauce.

Nutritional Information

- Calories: 522kcal
- Carbohydrates: 19g
- Protein: 36g
- Fat: 34g
- Cholesterol: 186mg
- Sodium: 191mg
- Potassium: 838mg
- Fiber: 4g
- Sugar: 8g
- Vitamin A: 1000IU
- Vitamin C: 17mg
- Calcium: 119mg
- Iron: 3mg

Healthy Egg Salad

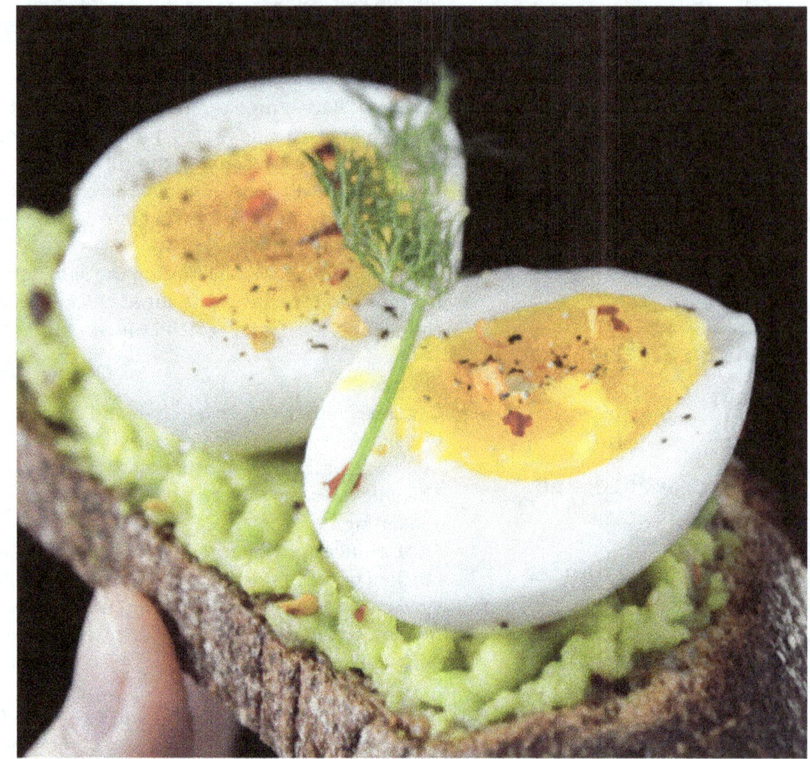

Prep time: 4 minutes
Cook time: 6 minutes
Servings: 4

Ingredients:

- 8 eggs hard boiled , chopped
- ¾ cup yogurt plain
- 2 tsp mustard spicy brown.

Procedure:

- Instant Pot
- Crack the eggs into an oven safe bowl that fits in the Instant Pot insert. Add 1 cup of water to the Instant Pot insert, then carefully lower the bowl of eggs to rest on the trivet. You can also hard-boil the eggs first, but this way is faster.
- Close the lid and turn the pressure valve to sealing. Cook on high pressure for 6 minutes, then let the pressure release naturally.
- Remove the lid and carefully lift the bowl from the Instant Pot. The bowl will be hot. Let the eggs cool to room temperature then slice the eggs into cubes.
- Gently mix in the yogurt, brown mustard, celery, paprika, parsley, and salt. Chill in the frigerator until ready to serve.
- Serve over a few leaves of lettuce and tomatoes to make a wrap.

- ½ cup celery chopped
- ½ tsp paprika
- 1 tsp parsley.

- Slow cooker
- Crack the eggs into an oven safe bowl that fits inside your slow cooker. Add 2 cups water to the slow cooker and place the bowl of eggs into the slow cooker. 8 eggs
- Cover the slow cooker with the lid. Cook the eggs on high heat for 1- 2 hours. When the yolks are set remove the bowl and let the eggs cool.
- Slice the eggs into cubes. Mix in the remaining ingredients. Chill the egg salad until ready to serve. Serve over leave of lettuce and slices of tomatoes.
- Oven
- Preheat oven to 350 degrees F. Crack the eggs into an oven safe bowl or pan. Bake the eggs for 20-25 minutes, until the yolks are cooked all the way through. 8 eggs
- Remove the pan from the oven and let it cool.
- Slice the eggs into cubes. Mix in the remaining ingredients. Chill the egg salad. Serve over leaves of lettuce and sliced of tomatoes when ready.

Nutritional Information

- Calories: 158kcal
- Carbohydrates: 3g
- Protein: 13g
- Fat: 10g
- Cholesterol: 333mg
- Sodium: 185mg
- Potassium: 225mg
- Fiber: 1g
- Sugar: 3g
- Vitamin A: 719IU
- Vitamin C: 1mg
- Calcium: 110mg
- Iron: 2mg

Healthy Dill Pickle Chicken Salad

**Prep time: 10 minutes
Cook time: 12 minutes
  Servings: 6**

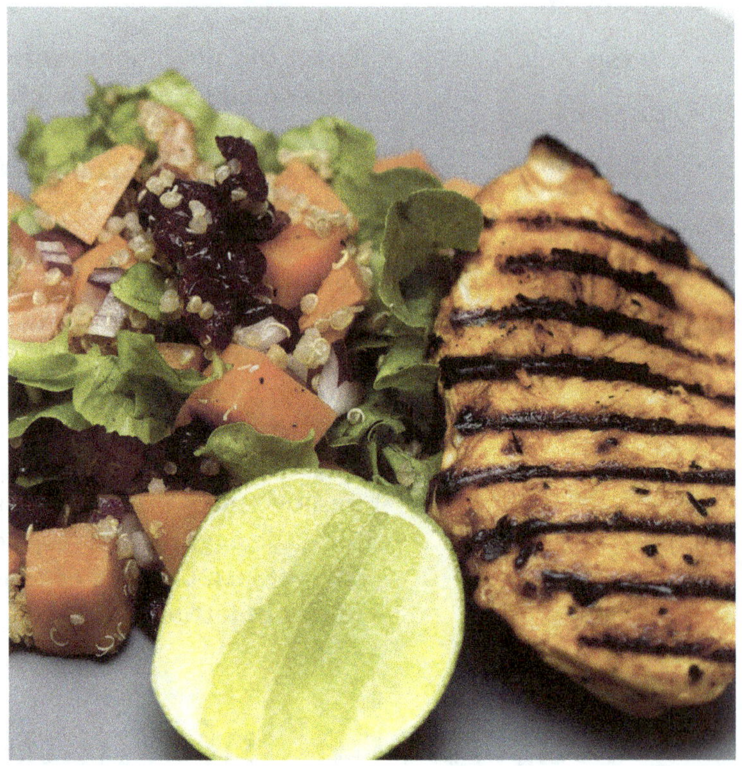

Ingredients:

- 1 pound chicken breast about 2 breasts
- 1/3 cup vinegar I use white
- 3/4 cup plain Greek yogurt
- 3/4 cup cottage cheese
- 1 tsp garlic
- 1 tsp black pepper

Procedure:

- Instant Pot
- Add the chicken and vinegar to the Instant Pot insert. 1 pound chicken breast, 1/3 cup vinegar
- Close the lid and turn the pressure valve to sealing. Cook the chicken on high pressure using the manual or pressure cook setting for 10-12 minutes. Let the pressure release naturally for at least 10 minutes before doing a quick release.
- In a food processor or blender, mix together the Greek yogurt, cottage cheese, garlic, and pepper until smooth.
- Remove the lid from the food processor or blender, then add the chicken to the food processor.
- Use the food processor or blender to shred the chicken and mix it with the sauce. It will only take about 5-15 seconds to shred the chicken.
- Take off the lid and remove the blade. Fold the chives, dill, parsley, and dill pickles into the dip. Garnish and serve with sliced veggies to dip.

55

- 1 tbsp fresh chives chopped (or 1 tsp dried)
- 1/2 tbsp fresh dill chopped (or 1/2 tsp dried)
- 1 tbsp fresh parsley chopped (or 1 tsp dried)
- 1 cup dill pickles chopped.

- Stove Top
- Add the chicken and vinegar to a sauce pan.
- Cover the sauce pan with a lid and cook the chicken on medium high temperature for 15-20 minutes until the chicken is cooked through.
- In a food processor or blender, mix together the Greek yogurt, cottage cheese, garlic, and pepper until smooth.
- Remove the lid from the food processor or blender, then add the chicken to the food processor. You may need to break the chicken breasts in half so that they fit.
- Use the food processor or blender to shred the chicken and mix it with the sauce. It will only take about 5-15 seconds to shred the chicken.
- Take off the lid and remove the blade. Fold the chives, dill, parsley, and dill pickles into the dip. Garnish and serve with sliced veggies to dip.
- Slow Cooker
- Add the chicken and vinegar to your slow cooker.
- Cover the slow cooker with the lid and cook the chicken on high heat for 2-3 hour, low heat for 4-5 hours.
- In a food processor or blender, mix together the Greek yogurt, cottage cheese, garlic, and pepper until smooth.
- Remove the lid from the food processor or blender then add the chicken to the food processor. You may need to break the chicken breasts in half so that they fit.
- Use the food processor or blender to shred the chicken and mix it with the sauce. It will only take about 5-15 seconds to shred the chicken.
- Take off the lid and remove the blade. Fold the chives, dill, parsley, and dill pickles into the dip. Garnish and serve with sliced veggies to dip.

Nutritional Information

- **Calories: 174kcal**
- **Fat :26g**
- **Cholestero:l 42mg**
- **Sodium: 649mg**
- **Total Carbohydrate: 14g**
- **Dietary Fiber: 4g**
- **Sugars: 6g**
- **Protein: 24g**

Fat- Free Dal Tadka

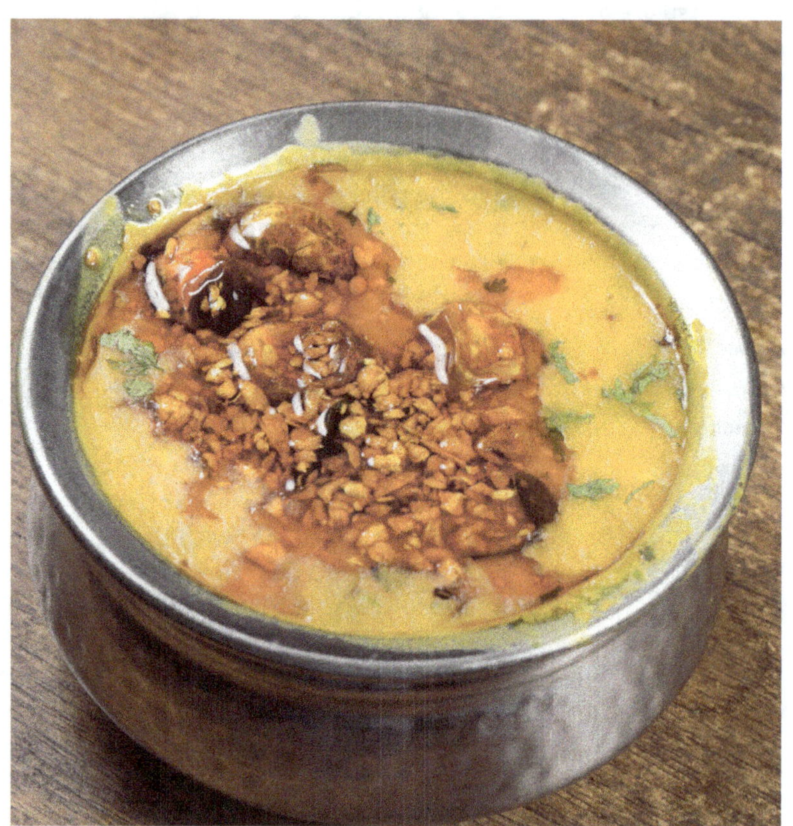

Prep time: 10 minutes
Cook time: 25 minutes

Servings: 6

Ingredients:

- 1/2 cup split red lentils
- 1/2 cup yellow moong dal
- 3 cups water
- 1 large tomato chopped
- 1/2 large onion chopped, set aside other half
- 3 cloves garlic minced
- 1 teaspoon ginger root minced.

Procedure:

- Put the lentils, water, and next 7 ingredients (through salt) into a pressure cooker and lock the lid. Cook at high pressure for 10 minutes. Allow pressure to drop naturally for 10 minutes and then do a quick-release.
- Open lid carefully and check to make sure lentils are tender. If not, continue to cook without pressure until lentils are fully cooked. Add garam masala and stir vigorously to make the lentils creamy. It should be a medium consistency, so add a little water if it's too thick. Keep warm.

57

- 1 teaspoon cumin seeds
- 1/2 teaspoon turmeric
- 1/2 teaspoon salt
- 1/2 teaspoon garam masala plus more to taste
- 1/2 large onion sliced
- 1/2 teaspoon red pepper flakes

- While the lentils are cooking, heat a small non-stick skillet. Add the onions and cook, stirring often, until they begin to brown. Add the red pepper flakes and cook until onions are softened and touched with brown.
- Check the seasoning of the lentils and add additional salt and garam masala to taste. Serve over rice and top each serving with the browned onions.

Nutritional Information

- Calories: 200kcal
- Fat: 0.8g
- Carbohydrates: 35g
- Protein: 15g
- Fiber: 7g
- Sodium: 500mg

Bolognese Sauce

**Prep time: 20 minutes
Cook time: 2 hours minutes
 Servings: 8**

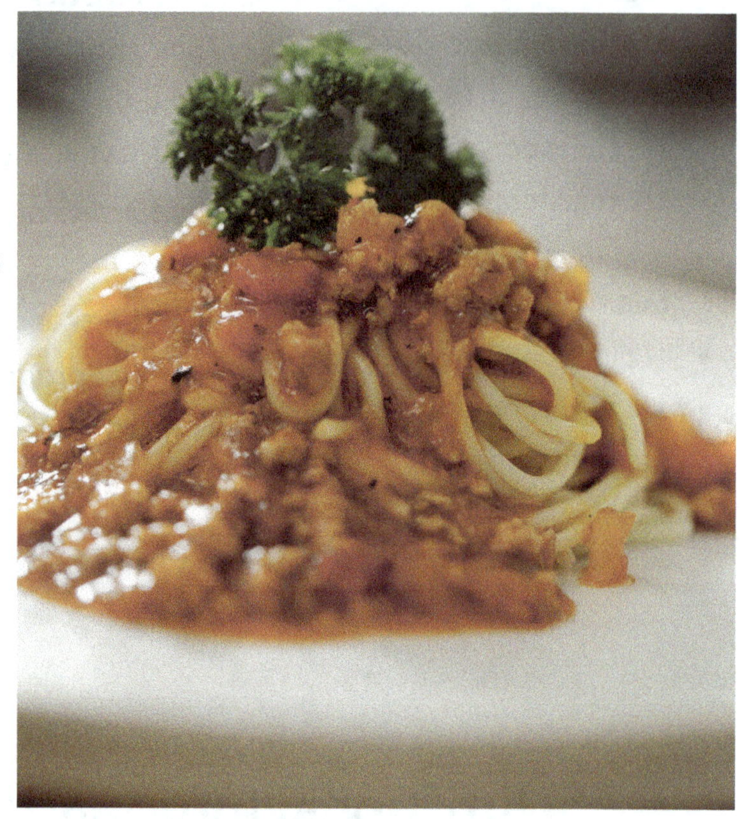

Ingredients:

- 1 lb 99% fat-free ground turkey breast
- 1 whole onion, diced fine
- 3 stalks celery, diced fine
- 3 whole carrots, diced fine
- 4 cloves garlic, minced
- 20 oz can diced tomatoes.

Procedure:

- In a large nonstick skillet, over medium heat saute onions, celery, carrots, and garlic until vegetables are tender. Use nonstick cooking spray as needed to prevent burning/sticking.
- Add ground turkey breast to the mixture and cook until no longer pink, mixing regularly.

- 2 cups fat-free beef broth
- 1/4 tsp fennel seed
- 1/8 tsp red pepper flakes
- 1/2 tsp black pepper
- 1/4 cup fresh basil, chopped
- 1/2 tsp salt
- Nonstick spray

- Add in fennel, red pepper flakes, black pepper, diced tomatoes, and beef broth. Mix well and simmer over medium heat for 10 minutes.
- Mix in fresh basil and salt to taste.
- Continue cooking for additional 5-10 minutes or until flavors have melded together well.
- Serve over favorite pasta.

Nutritional Information

- Calories: 300kcal
- Fat: 15g
- Carbohydrates: 20g
- Protein: 25g
- Fiber: 4g
- Sodium: 800mg

Spicy Chicken Zoodle Soup

Prep time: 15 minutes
Cook time: 25 minutes
Servings: 6

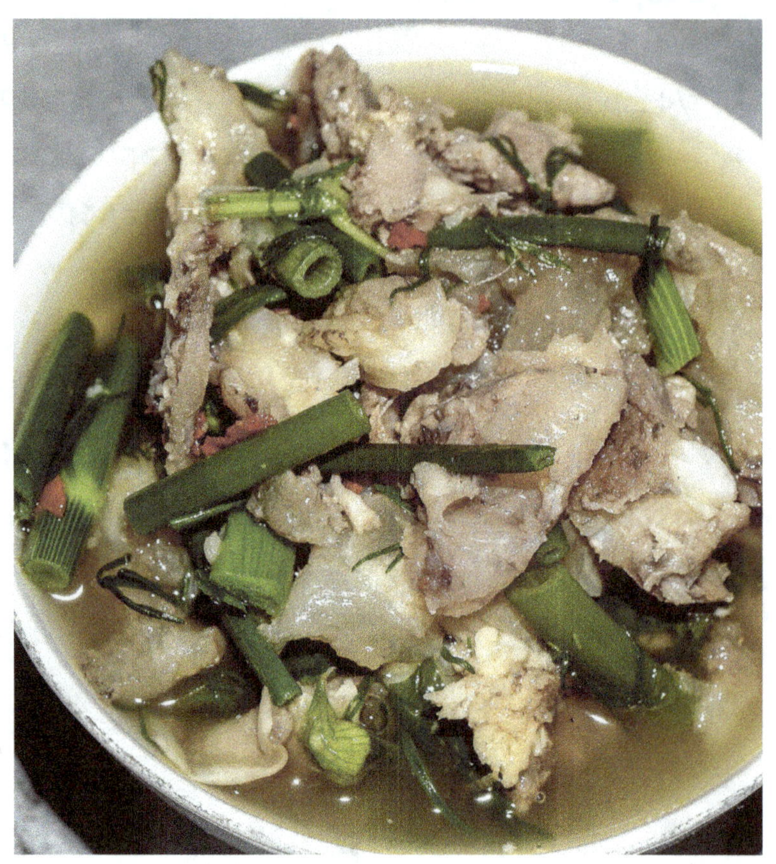

Ingredients:

- 2 tbsp (30 ml) avocado oil or olive oil
- 1 medium yellow onion, diced
- 1 lb (450 g) boneless skinless chicken breast, cut into bite-size pieces
- 1 tsp Kosher salt
- ½ tsp ground black pepper

Procedure:

- Heat a large stock pot to medium heat. Once hot, add the oil and sauté the onion for 3 minutes.
- Place the chicken, salt and pepper into the pot. Sauté with the onion for another 3 to 4 minutes. Add the celery, carrots, chicken broth and hot sauce. Bring to a boil, reduce the heat to a simmer and add the zucchini noodles.

61

- 3 stalks celery, diced (about 1 cup
- 4 large carrots, peeled and diced (about 1 cup
- 40 oz (1.2 L) chicken broth
- ¼–½ cup (60–120 ml) buffalo hot sauce (see note)
- 3 cups (420 g) zucchini noodles
- ¼ cup (4 g) fresh cilantro

- Let simmer for another 5 to 7 minutes before serving. Garnish with fresh cilantro.

Nutritional Information

- Calories: 300kcal
- Protein: 30g
- Carbohydrates: 15g
- Fat: 13g
- Fiber: 4g

Grilled Picnic Chicken

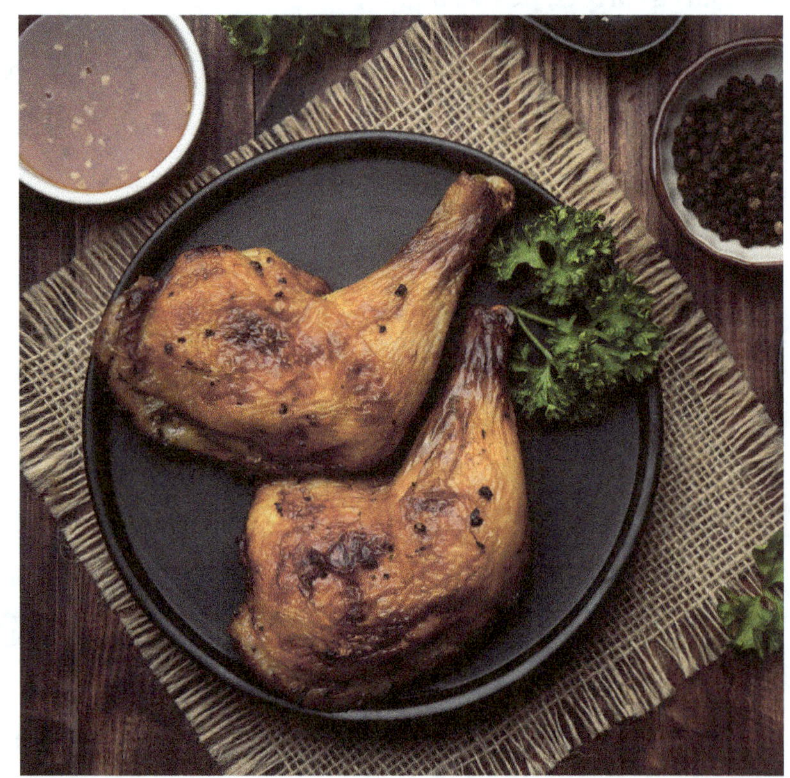

Prep time: 10 minutes
Cook time: 25 minutes
Servings: 4

Ingredients:

- 1½ cups white vinegar
- ¾ cup canola oil
- 6 Tbsp water
- 4½ tsp salt
- 1½ tsp poultry seasoning.

Procedure:

- In a bowl, combine white vinegar, canola oil, water, salt, poultry seasoning, garlic powder and pepper. Remove 1 cup for basting; cover and refrigerate.
- Pour remaining marinade into a large shallow dish; add chicken. Turn to coat; refrigerate for 4 hours or overnight, turning once or twice.

- ¾ tsp garlic powder
- ¾ tsp pepper
- 3 (to 4-lb) broiler/fryer chickens, cut into pieces

- Drain chicken, discarding marinade in dish. Grill chicken, uncovered, over medium heat for 15 minutes on each side. Baste with reserved marinade. Grill chicken 10 to 20 minutes longer or until juices run clear, turning and basting several times.

Nutritional Information

- Calories: 300kcal
- Protein: 30g
- Carbohydrates: 10g
- Fat: 15g
- Fiber: 0g

Slow Cooker Tex Mex Chicken And Beans

Prep time: 15 minutes
Cook time: 8 hours
Servings: 4

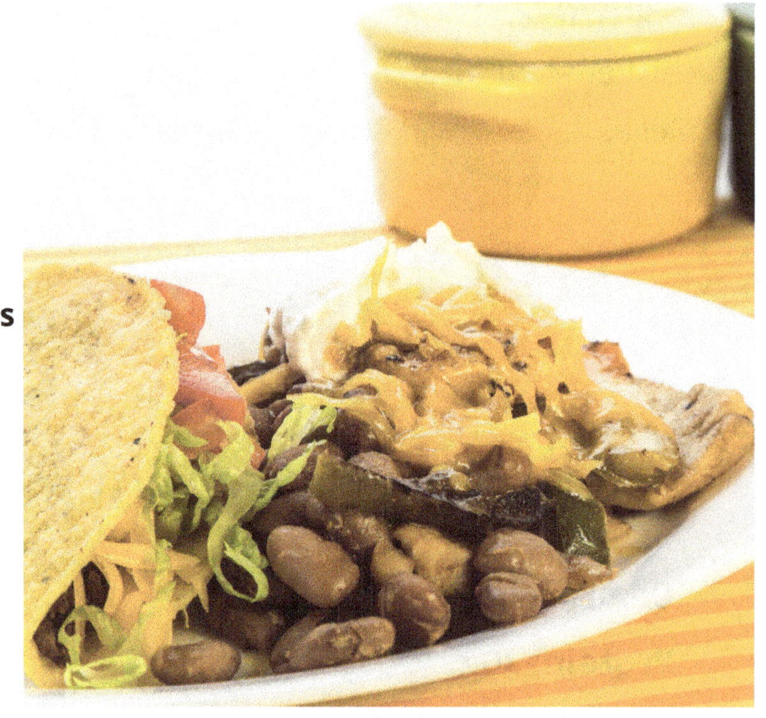

Ingredients:

- 1 cup dried pinto beans, rinsed and soaked in water for at least a couple of hours
- One 16 ounce jar mild or medium salsa
- 2 tablespoons chopped canned chipotle in adobo sauce

Procedure:

- In a 5 to 6 quart slow cooker, stir together drained beans, salsa, chiles, flour, 1 cup water, onion and bell pepper.
- Cover and cook on low heat for 4 hours. Season chicken generously with salt and pepper; arrange on top of bean mixture, add another cup of water, and cook on low heat for 4 more hours.

- 2 tablespoons all purpose flour
- 1 medium red onion, chopped
- 1 medium red bell pepper, seeds and ribs removed, chopped
- coarse salt and freshly ground black pepper
- 1½ pounds boneless, skinless chicken
- ¼ cup chopped fresh cilantro.

- Shred chicken, and stir.
- Serve over brown rice, or inside flour tortillas to make tacos (not included in the nutritional). Garnish with cilantro and additional desired toppings.

Nutritional Information

- Calories: 440kcal
- Carbohydrates: 46g
- Protein: 46g
- Fat: 8g
- Cholesterol: 162mg
- Sodium: 1290mg
- Potassium: 1494mg
- Fiber: 11g,
- Sugar: 8g
- Vitamin A: 1960IU
- Vitamin C: 46mg
- Calcium: 111mg
- Iron: 5mg

Slow Cooker Butternut Squash Soup

Prep time: 15 minutes
Cook time: 8 hours
Servings: 6

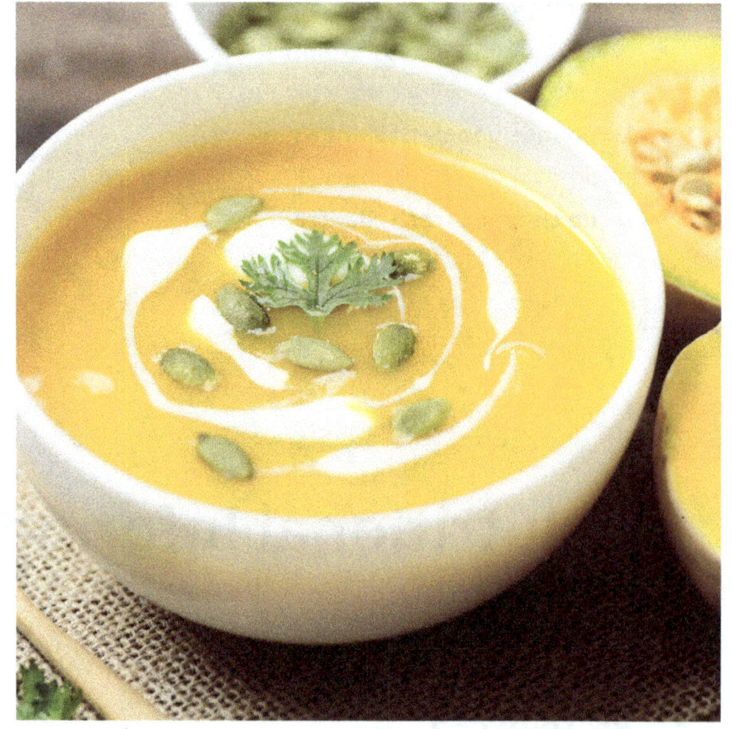

Ingredients:

- 2 butternut squash, peeled and chopped
- 1 onion, chopped
- 4 cloves garlic, minced
- 1 carrot, chopped
- 2 apples, chopped (peeled)
- 2 cups vegetable broth

Procedure:

- everything to the slow cooker except the coconut milk. Cook on low for 6-8 hours until squash is completely tender.
- Add the coconut milk to the slow cooker. Use an immersion blender to blend to a smooth consistency. You could also use a regular blender and blend in batches. Taste and season with salt and pepper.

67

- 1 tsp kosher salt
- 1 sprig fresh sage
- 1/4 tsp nutmeg
- 1/4 tsp black pepper
- 1/8 tsp cayenne pepper
- 3/4 cup canned coconut
  milk

Nutritional Information

- Calories: 196kcal
- Fat 8g
- Cholesterol: 0mg
- Sodium: 726mg
- Total Carbohydrate: 35g
- Dietary Fiber: 6g
- Sugars: 13g